# FIGHTING FIT

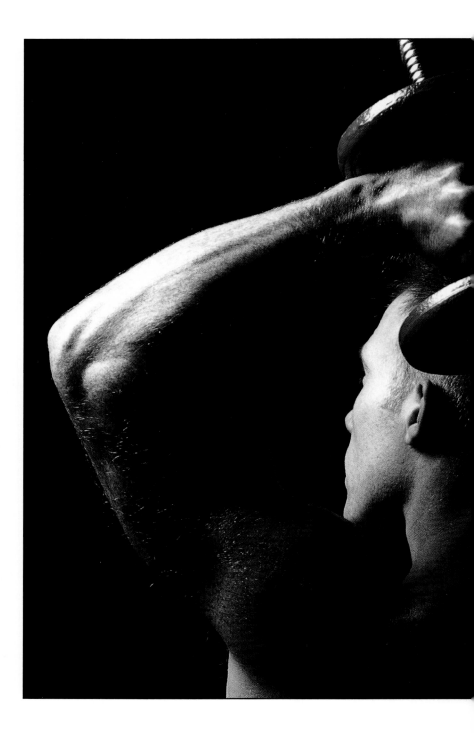

MAN ALIVE

# FIGHTING FIT

## Toni Battison

MACMILLAN ◆ USA

Conceived, edited, and designed by
MARSHALL EDITIONS
170 Piccadilly
London W1V 9DD

*Copyright © Marshall Editions Developments Limited 1997*

First published in the U.S.A. in 1997
by Macmillan Publishing Company, a division of Macmillan, Inc.

**MACMILLAN**
**A Simon & Schuster Macmillan Company**
**1633 Broadway**
**New York, NY 10019**

Library of Congress Cataloging-in-Publication Data

Battison, Toni.
        Fighting fit / Toni Battison.
                p. cm. — (Man alive)
        Includes index.
        ISBN  0–02–861505–0
    1.  Physical fitness for men.
    I.  Title.  II. Series: Man alive (New York. N.Y.)
    RA777.8.B38  1997
    613.7'0449—dc20                                          96–9651
                                                             CIP

10  9  8  7  6  5  4  3  2  1

*Originated in Singapore by Classicscan*
*Printed and bound in Portugal by Printer Portugesa*

| | |
|---|---|
| **Editor** | Jonathan Hilton |
| **Art editor** | Vicky Holmes |
| **Photographer** | Laura Wickenden |
| **DTP editors** | Mary Pickles, Kate Waghorn |
| **Copy editors** | Jolika Feszt, Maggi McCormick |
| **Indexer** | Judy Batchelor |
| **Managing editor** | Lindsay McTeague |
| **Production editor** | Emma Dixon |
| **Art director** | Sean Keogh |
| **Editorial director** | Sophie Collins |
| **Production** | Bob Christie |

# CONTENTS

# WHAT IS FITNESS?

*In basic terms, being fit means being physically active at a level that allows you to cope with the demands of life without undue stress.*

Whether you want to train for a particular sport, improve your overall level of fitness, simply feel better about yourself, or achieve a body that looks good and performs efficiently, you must consider your present level of fitness before you embark on any program of exercise. Fitness is about strong, toned muscles; efficient heart and lungs; and flexible joints. Like a car, a well-tuned body will always provide you with that little extra burst of energy when it is really needed but, again like a car, your body must be kept tuned with regular exercise or it will soon revert to its less efficient ways.

Fitness, though, is a relative state, and levels vary across a whole range of sports and other types of activity. A swimmer's fitness, for example, would be a different type of fitness from that of a runner.

## FITNESS FACTORS

There are several factors that help determine the personal level of fitness you should aspire to:
- age
- weight
- ability
- body maintenance
(do you smoke, eat well?)
- how active you have been in the past
- the type of activity that you currently undertake
- any existing injury.

## WHY DO YOU WANT TO BE FIT?

Whatever your reasons for wanting to be fit, you will have a better chance of sticking to your program if you keep your goals in the front of your mind. You are bound to feel a bit stiff at first, but you can look forward to:
- improved stamina, suppleness, and strength
- better general health
- increased metabolic rate
- reduction in body weight
- increased self-esteem
- changes in your social life
- increased pleasure and a sense of achievement
- reduced anxiety and tension.

## WHOLE BODY FITNESS

No matter what your personal goal is – whether to improve your overall health, increase your skill in a particular sport, or generally feel good about your body image – you should aim to achieve it in a holistic way. The object is to look and feel better, not to

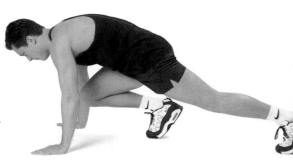

overdevelop one set of muscles or go home exhausted at the end of the day.

Whole body fitness will improve your metabolic process (the rate at which your body burns calories for energy) and increase your stamina, suppleness, and strength. As you strive for personal fitness, keep these three S's firmly in mind – they are the key factors in achieving endurance, power, and flexibility.

**Stamina** is about keeping going. It is poor stamina that is usually responsible for making you tire easily and feel unfit. Stamina-increasing exercises are clearly vital if you are training for a marathon or long-distance cycling. However, stamina is just as beneficial for ordinary activities, such as climbing stairs.

**Suppleness** helps you to bend, stretch, and twist your body, whatever your level of activity. A supple body will improve your agility in the gym, and equally, it will help you when you need to change a tire.

**Strength** is linked to muscular endurance and power, and is vital when you need to exert force for pushing, pulling, or lifting. All sportsmen must have strength and power, but strength is also useful for carrying heavy shopping bags.

### KEEP IT UP

The key message is to keep exercising. Being fit is a continuous process; stop, even for a few weeks, and you will soon be back where you started. A few hours of action a week is not a high price to pay for health – and it can be fun.

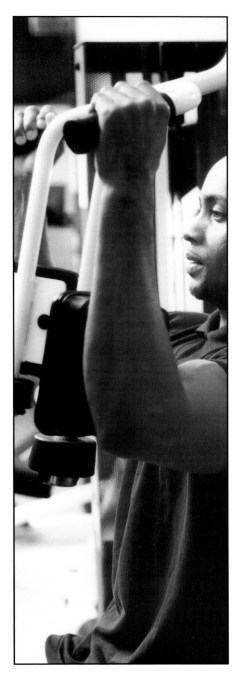

# DEVISING A FITNESS PROGRAM

*As soon as exercise becomes a part of your daily routine, you will begin to reap the benefits of improved health and general well being. With a healthier body you will look better, feel better, and have more fun.*

The question you are probably asking is: how do I get started? You can start right now with some small changes – even 10 minutes of brisk exercise each day will have an immediate effect. Simple lifestyle changes, such as using your car less and walking up a few flights of stairs instead of taking the elevator, will start to increase your stamina while you get on with the next stage: devising a planned fitness program. Here are some general points to consider:

◆ Build up your program slowly if you haven't exercised recently.

◆ Fit your program into your normal life for a better chance of sticking to it in the long term.

◆ Reduce the risk of injury by using the right equipment, clothes, and warm-up/cool-down routines.

◆ Know your limits – you are aiming to be fit, not Superman.

◆ Share your exercise with a partner – it adds to the fun.

◆ Work your muscles regularly– there are no short cuts to fitness.

◆ Choose the exercises that are right for you – pleasure, convenience, and cost are the key words to remember.

◆ Vary your program – don't let boredom get in the way of progress.

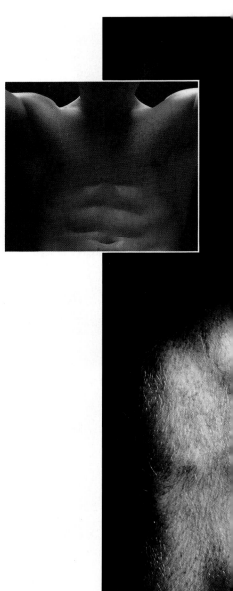

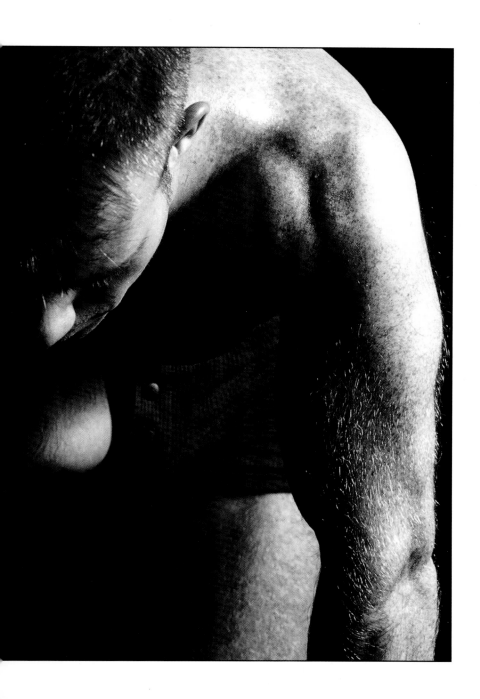

# HOW FIT ARE YOU?

*Measure your fitness level before deciding on the best form of exercise for you.*

If you have a sedentary lifestyle, you need to adopt a different approach to getting fit from the regular exerciser's.

### LOW FITNESS LEVEL
*Less than 30 minutes of moderate physical activity a week.*
You need to become steadily more active by taking a little more exercise each day. If time is short, fit exercise into your routine. Move around more vigorously so you feel warm and slightly out of breath; walk up stairs and escalators; walk briskly or bicycle to work. Aim for 60 minutes of moderate exercise spread over a week.

### MEDIUM FITNESS LEVEL
*30 minutes of moderate physical activity, up to five times a week.*
A health club or gym might suit you. You are probably interested enough to benefit from a personal exercise plan, and you should aim to increase from moderate to energetic exercise for up to 2½ hours a week.

### HIGH FITNESS LEVEL
*30 minutes of moderate physical activity, at least 5 times a week.*
Increase from moderate to energetic activity for at least 2½ hours a week and guard against boredom by trying a new sport or using a personal trainer.

### BODY TESTS
If you wish to embark on a program of vigorous exercise, a gym or health club will advise you on how to start. All gyms offer fitness tests to check your:
◆ overall fitness rating
◆ levels of stamina, suppleness, and strength
◆ body fat percentages.
Alternatively, you could carry out some basic tests at home, perhaps with the help of a partner.
**Pulse rate** Measuring your pulse rate during exercise will keep you within safe exercise levels for burning fat and getting fitter. Your pulse is most easily felt on the inner side of your wrist on the same side as your thumb (radial pulse), or at the side of the neck, under the jaw (carotid pulse). You will need a watch or clock with a second hand. Check your pulse rate after sitting quietly for about 15 minutes. This is known as your resting pulse rate. The heart beats about 70 times every minute in the averagely fit person.

| Resting pulse rate (beats per minute) | Level of fitness |
|---|---|
| 50–59 | Excellent (trained athlete) |
| 60–69 | Good |
| 70–79 | Fair |
| 80 or more | Poor |

When exercising, you need to keep your heart working at a safe level. This is most easily done by taking your pulse over a 10-second period and making sure that it stays within the 10-second pulse range for your age, as shown on the chart below.

| Age | 10-second pulse range |
|-----|----------------------|
| 20 | 20–27 |
| 25 | 20–26 |
| 30 | 19–25 |
| 35 | 19–25 |
| 40 | 18–24 |
| 50 | 17–23 |
| 60 | 16–21 |
| 65 | 16–21 |
| 70 | 15–20 |

Take your 10-second pulse every 10 minutes while exercising. If you are unfit, make sure your pulse stays at the lower end of your range at first, and slowly work toward the upper end. If at any time your pulse rate goes higher than it should, stop exercising and walk around slowly until it drops. When you restart, take it easy.

Try taking your pulse a minute after stopping exercise; the quicker it falls, the fitter you are. After a 10-minute rest, your heart rate should have fallen to below 100 beats per minute.

**Muscle tests** Muscles vary in their potential for development. The rule is: the longer the muscle, the more it can be developed. Stand on the toes of one leg and check where your calf muscle ends. The closer it is to your heel, the more room there is for muscle development. Do the same with your upper arm. Make a tight fist and check how close your biceps are to the elbow.

**Suppleness test** You can assess suppleness by trying to touch your toes. It is important to warm up first (*see pp. 26–27*) so you don't damage your hamstrings. You will also get a truer result. Sit on the ground with your legs together. Keep your back straight and, as you inhale, lift your arms above your head. As you exhale, lean forward and stretch your fingers toward your toes. Keep your back straight and don't stretch your neck forward. Do this three times and take the best stretch as your measurement.

◆ Up to 5 in (13 cm) from toes: Poor
◆ Almost or touching toes: Fair
◆ Reach past toes: Good.

**Stamina/fitness test** Try this test to check your fitness at the start of your program and again after training for two months. The rating will depend on your age and how active you are generally. Use it as a basic guide only.

◆ Accurately measure how long it takes you to cover 1 mile (1.5 km).
◆ Walk or run, using a combination if you need to, to cover the measured distance as quickly as possible without becoming uncomfortably breathless.
◆ Stop if you experience any pain or serious discomfort.

| Minutes for 1 mile (1.5 km) | Stamina/ fitness level |
|-----------------------------|------------------------|
| 20 or more | Very unfit |
| 15–20 | Unfit |
| 12–15 | Fairly fit |
| 10–12 | Fit |
| 10 or less | Very fit |

# AIMS AND OBJECTIVES

*Before you start a fitness program, it helps to formulate a clear idea of what you want*
*achieve. Look at the list below and check the boxes that reflect how you feel.*

**PHYSICAL**
**I want to:**

- [ ] Have more energy
- [ ] Improve my heart and lung function
- [x] Have more flexible joints
- [x] Have less body fat and firmer muscles
- [x] Improve my posture and body shape
- [ ] Improve my sleep patterns
- [ ] Increase my stamina
- [ ] Become better coordinated
- [ ] Reduce my risk of injury

**PSYCHOLOGICAL**
**I want to:**

- [ ] Reduce my stress and anxiety levels
- [ ] Increase my sense of achievement
- [x] Feel good about myself
- [ ] Have the opportunity to let off steam
- [ ] Feel ready to meet new challenges
- [ ] Set aside time for myself
- [ ] Use exercise as an aid to giving up smoking
- [x] Feel better about my body shape

**SOCIAL**
**I want to:**

- [x] Meet new people and make new friends
- [ ] Enjoy being active
- [ ] Use exercise as a status symbol
- [ ] Improve my work image
- [ ] Try new challenges
- [ ] Learn new skills
- [x] Improve my sex life
- [ ] Find an alternative to going to the bar after work
- [ ] Support environmental issues by using my car less

**KEEPING UP THE MOTIVATION**

Many people who decide to become fitter start off with the best of intentions, but somehow other things get in the way. Do any of these comments sound familiar?

*"I'm always busy, so I don't need to do more exercise."*

*"I'm not the sporty type."*

*"Life is too full already to visit a gym or jog around the block."*

*"I start off well, but then I slip back into lazy habits."*

*"I am too tired to exercise; I need to relax."*

*"My body isn't good enough to show in public."*

*"I don't know how to get started."*

*"I have a disability."*

*"Right now, work is more important than exercise."*

If you recognize yourself here, then think positively and turn your good intentions into real action. Motivation is the key. Use the SMART formula to help set realistic objectives. Above all, set goals that suit your needs – that you believe you can manage and will enjoy. Be flexible – it is not a sin if your schedule wavers a little. Don't be influenced by other people's goals – theirs will be different – and don't let them talk you into believing in the "No Pain, No Gain" philosophy. Exercise need not hurt to produce results.

## SMART formula

**S**pecific: I will choose a routine based on my needs.
**M**easurable: I will exercise X times per week.
**A**ction: I will join a gym or swim three times a week.
**R**ealistic: I will set sensible goals.
**T**ime-related: I will review my progress at the end of one/six months.

### FITTING THE PROGRAM INTO YOUR SCHEDULE

If you are always flying off on business trips that confine you to a hotel room between meetings and working lunches, it may not be possible to stick to a regular routine or visit a gym. But don't use this as an excuse to abandon your fitness program.

To maintain a fit body, the average person needs to exercise for about 90 minutes a week. The good news is that it does not have to be in large chunks. If your time is limited, short, regular bursts of intense exercise – for example, nine sets of 10 minutes each – are excellent. If you can set aside more time, better still. The important point is that you exercise regularly. Have a tone-up session in the office, or make use of idle time in your hotel room.

◆ Look at your schedule and plan your exercise around meetings and conferences.
◆ Explore your surroundings with a brisk daily walk.
◆ Team up with a colleague and do some shared exercises (*see pp. 22–23*).
◆ Jog around the block.

◆ Invest in a portable set of basic gym equipment, available from sporting goods stores.

### PLANNING A PROGRAM

Plan a 30-minute routine for when you have more time available for exercise. Choose from the menu below to devise a varied program that will hold your interest.

**Warm up:** 5 minutes (*see pp. 26–27*)
**Aerobics/Stamina:** 15 minutes
  Brisk walking – use a park or walk around the block.
  Swimming (if the hotel has a pool) – aim to keep moving and vary your strokes.
  Jogging – distance about 1–1½ miles (1.5–2.5 km).
  Skipping – this can be exhausting if you have not skipped recently, so include rests if needed.
**Strength**
  Inner thigh raises (*see p. 42*)
  Hamstring curls (*see p. 43*)
  Push-ups (*see pp. 50–51*). Choose the type suitable for your ability
  Triceps dips (*see p. 48*)
  Single arm crunches (*see p. 55*)
  Twists (*see p. 55*)
**Suppleness**
  Quad stretches (*see pp. 56–57*)
  Upper calf stretches (*see p. 57*)
  Neck stretches (*see p. 61*)
  Forearm stretches (*see p. 61*)
  Total body stretches (*see p. 66*)
**Cool down:** 5 minutes (*see pp. 28–29*)
  Slow walk or swim or finish with some of the gentle stretches from the suppleness range.

# WHAT'S BEST FOR ME?

*How to choose the best exercise for your lifestyle and level of fitness.*

The easiest approach if you are a beginner is to concentrate on building up your stamina with aerobic exercise, such as walking and swimming, and to include some basic stretching exercises to increase your suppleness. Keep the strength and endurance activities to a minimum until you are ready to expand your range (*see chart on p. 33*).

When you plan your program, there are three so-called FIT variables over which you have some control:
**Frequency** – how often you exercise
**Intensity** – how hard you exercise
**Time** – how long you exercise.
If you can devote only a limited amount of time to exercise, in order to move up the fitness "scale" you will have to work progressively harder by increasing the intensity of your effort rather than the duration.

## HOW LONG SHOULD I SPEND?

There is no easy answer to this question, since it depends on your personal goals. If, for example, 10 minutes of exercise a day will increase your basic fitness, then 30 minutes a day will have a greater effect. However, when you increase the intensity of your effort, you also need to take into account the amount of muscle you are using, since basically the more muscles you work, the greater the benefit within a fixed time ratio. The table below helps to explain this effect.

| Exercise for same effect | Minimum time required |
|---|---|
| Walking briskly | 40 minutes |
| Cycling | 25 minutes |
| Swimming | 20 minutes |
| Jogging | 15 minutes |
| Rowing | 15 minutes |

### TARGET TRAINING ZONE

You should always exercise within safe limits. The graph opposite will help you to judge what is right for you. The points to remember are:
◆ Your maximum heart rate is set at 220 beats per minute minus your age.
◆ During warm up, increase your pulse from its resting rate to 40–60 percent of its maximum.
◆ As you exercise, aim for 60–80 percent of your maximum heart rate.

The golden rule is: if it hurts, stop. If at any time you become so breathless that you can't speak, develop chest tightness or pain, or feel dizzy or unwell, stop immediately and seek medical advice.

To use the graph, look along the horizontal axis for your age and check against the heartbeat rate on the vertical axis. After warming up, you should aim to exercise within the highlighted band.

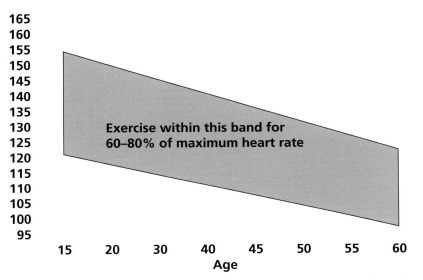

165
160
155
150
145
140
135
130
125
120
115
110
105
100
95

**Exercise within this band for
60–80% of maximum heart rate**

15  20  30  40  45  50  55  60

**Age**

PROGRAM PLANNING

You need to be realistic about how fit you really are, since most people overestimate their fitness. Don't attempt any activities that feel beyond your capacity. Consult your doctor if you have a heart condition, high blood pressure, asthma, bronchitis, diabetes, arthritis, joint pains, back problems, or if you are recovering from an illness or operation. Start with moderate activities and build up gradually.

The chart below shows how this can be done over a 12-week period, mixing levels of activity and working toward three 30- to 40-minute sessions a week. All the activities are designed to improve stamina and, together with a controlled diet, will help with weight management. Choose any activities from the stamina section. The times given do not include warming up and cooling down (*see pp. 26–29*), both of which are essential.

|  | Session one | Session two | Session three |
|---|---|---|---|
| **Weeks 1–3** | A x 10 mins | B x 10 mins | A x 15 mins |
| **Weeks 4–6** | A x 20 mins | B x 15 mins | B x 15 mins |
| **Weeks 7–9** | B x 20 mins | B x 20 mins | C x 20 mins |
| **Weeks 10–12** | B x 30 mins | C x 20 mins | B x 30 mins |

KEY
A  gentle activity: 50–60% of maximum heart rate
B  moderate activity: 60–70% of maximum heart rate
C  aerobic activity: 70–80% of maximum heart rate

# THE MAJOR MUSCLE GROUPS

*Muscles are composed of specialized tissue, or fibers, that contract and relax to help you to perform sequences of movements.*

Although the size and strength of your individual muscles have a bearing on your level of fitness, you don't need a deep understanding of these factors to exercise effectively. But it may be useful to know the main muscle groups shown here and on pages 18–19.

Muscles require a constant supply of blood from which they extract nutrients. This process takes place through the cardiovascular and respiratory systems, and is called aerobic (with oxygen) action. As you train and increase the demands on your heart and other muscles, the whole process becomes more efficient.

The body's cells – including muscle cells – store energy in the form of the chemical adenosine triphosphate (ATP).

Energy is released when the cells split the high-energy bonds of ATP. In aerobic activity you will breathe hard, so as much oxygen as possible reacts with glucose to make more ATP.

In anaerobic activity, your ATP reserves allow your muscles to work for about 10 seconds without oxygen; if you continue such activity, the body produces another 10 seconds' worth of ATP using phosphate creatine (PC). After this, any further energy comes from glycogen, in a reaction that has lactic acid as a byproduct. Among the side effects are painful muscles and possible cramps. When you stop the anaerobic activity, after a sprint, say, you will be out of breath until your body has replenished your ATP stores.

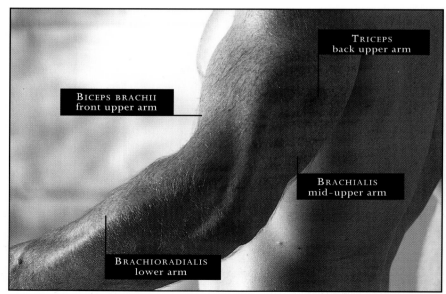

TRICEPS
back upper arm

BICEPS BRACHII
front upper arm

BRACHIALIS
mid-upper arm

BRACHIORADIALIS
lower arm

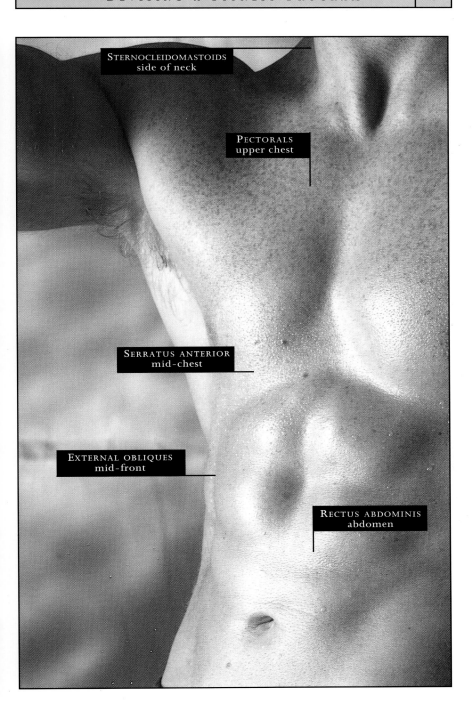

STERNOCLEIDOMASTOIDS
side of neck

PECTORALS
upper chest

SERRATUS ANTERIOR
mid-chest

EXTERNAL OBLIQUES
mid-front

RECTUS ABDOMINIS
abdomen

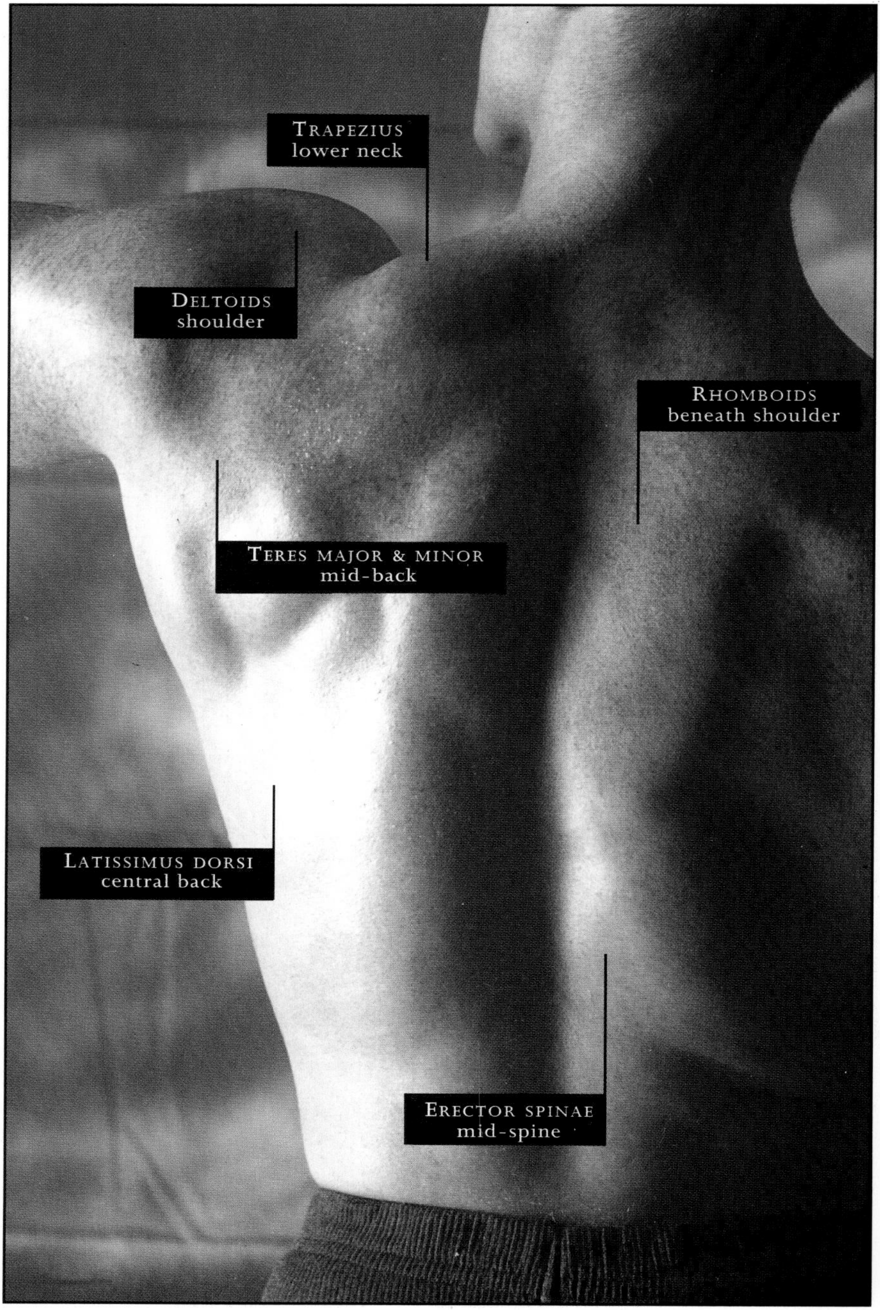

TRAPEZIUS
lower neck

DELTOIDS
shoulder

RHOMBOIDS
beneath shoulder

TERES MAJOR & MINOR
mid-back

LATISSIMUS DORSI
central back

ERECTOR SPINAE
mid-spine

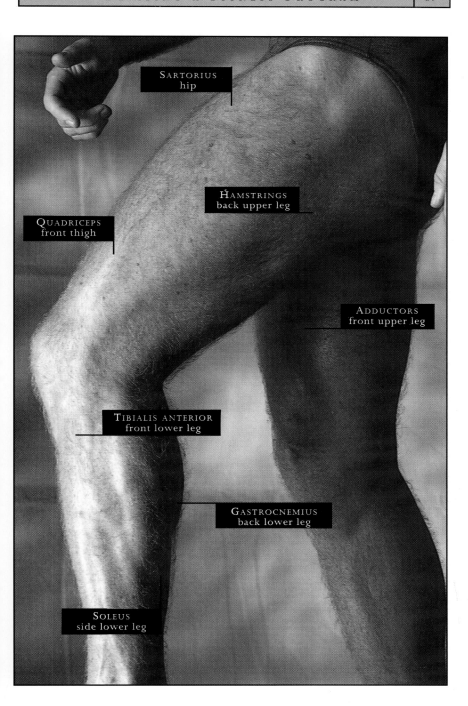

SARTORIUS
hip

HAMSTRINGS
back upper leg

QUADRICEPS
front thigh

ADDUCTORS
front upper leg

TIBIALIS ANTERIOR
front lower leg

GASTROCNEMIUS
back lower leg

SOLEUS
side lower leg

# WHAT WILL I NEED?

*For most activities and home exercise, you won't need to spend much for equipment, clothes, and footwear.*

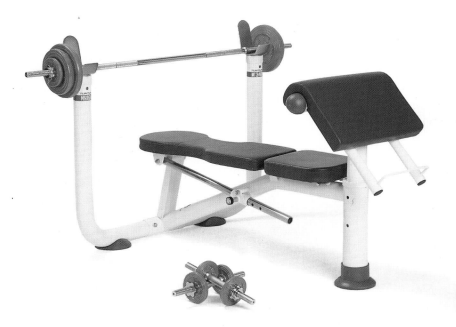

Don't rush to the store in a wave of enthusiasm to buy the latest fashion in sportswear without first checking your needs. Ask yourself: what do I have already; what activity do I plan to specialize in; how often will my clothes need to be washed; will I need to keep one set at home and another at work? Listen to the advice offered by the clerks in the sporting goods stores; they should value your business and not encourage you to buy unnecessary equipment.

## EQUIPMENT

If you plan to exercise mainly at home, you will need to invest in certain equipment. Good-quality items can be expensive, so start with smaller pieces and gradually build up. Questions to ask include: what can I afford; what is essential; is the equipment stable and adjustable; how often will I use it; is it safe to use alone; do I know how to use it or do I need training; is it maintenance-free; are there guarantees?

Choose from the following items for beginner to intermediate levels: watch with a second hand, mat, personal alarm (for jogging), step platform – one that fits your whole foot), skipping rope, exercise bike, rowing machine, bench with rack, treadmill, wrist/ankle weights, and dumbbells. For advanced levels, consider adding bar weights and a trampoline.

## CLOTHES
Choose comfortable, loose-fitting clothes made of fabrics that allow heat and moisture to escape. For indoor work, you will need two sets of shorts and T-shirts, plus a tracksuit and sweatshirt. For outdoor activity, consider hooded sweatshirts, waterproof clothing, a hat, T-shirts, and gloves. Several pairs of sports socks are an essential investment. Look for neat seams and the correct size in a synthetic/natural-fiber mix.

## SHOES
For any exercise, you need a good pair of shoes with thick, cushioned soles and heels to prevent jarring. They should be wide and long enough for comfort, bearing in mind that your feet will swell during exercise and that sports socks are usually quite thick. Shoes should also have good arch support and strong heel cups.

For a varied program, you may need more than one pair. For aerobics combined with general sports, go for cross trainers; for walking, choose shoes with stability, shock absorbency and flexibility; shoes for tennis and squash need strong toes and lateral support straps; and running and jogging shoes need to be durable, be shock absorbent, support your heels, and have the correct sole for the running surface. Visit a sports store when your feet are warm and have them check the shape of your instep.

## UNDERWEAR
Choose cotton material that is well cut in the crotch to avoid abrasion; briefs instead of jockstraps are fine. Choose separate briefs rather than those built into shorts. These tend to be synthetic and not as comfortable.

## BELTS
These should be necessary only if you exercise with heavy weights, which you are unlikely to do unless you need to build up considerable strength for an event or you are a serious weightlifter. Belts support the weaker muscles to allow the stronger ones to perform at their best. They are usually worn around the abdominal area, where they help to contract the muscles, increase pressure, and support the spine. A belt should be tight, but with enough room to allow you to breathe deeply. Get advice when choosing a belt, since the correct width is important.

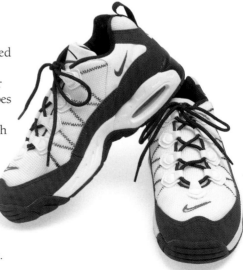

# STRETCHING WITH A PARTNER

*The two major advantages of working with a partner are that you can increase the intensity of a stretch and that you can hold it for longer.*

### SEATED GROIN STRETCHES
◆ Sit on the floor with your back straight, head in line with your spine, and your abdominals pulled in. Relax your shoulders.
◆ Place the soles of your feet squarely together and allow your knees to drop apart.
◆ Your partner should now kneel behind you and place both hands on the inside of your knees or thighs, depending on which is easier to reach.
◆ When you are both comfortable, ask your partner to press down on your inner knees, easing your legs toward the floor. Hold and repeat exercise.

You need to trust your partner if this form of stretching is to work. You are relinquishing control of the movement and, therefore, run the risk of overstretching and straining your muscles. If you are not relaxed, your muscles will not stretch, and it is vital not to force. Start with small movements and then build up gradually. If you feel any discomfort, stop at once.

**SEATED GROIN STRETCHES**
MUSCLES WORKED: ADDUCTORS
HOLD: 8–30 SECONDS
GOOD FOR: CYCLING, RUNNING

**SHOULDER STRETCHES**
MUSCLES WORKED: PECTORALS, ANTERIOR DELTOIDS
HOLD: 8–30 SECONDS
GOOD FOR: SWIMMING, TENNIS

### SHOULDER STRETCHES
◆ Sit on the floor with your back straight, head in line with your spine, and your abdominals in. Stretch your legs out in front, keeping your knees and feet together.
◆ Raise both arms over your head. Your partner should take your wrists and put one knee in the middle of your back to keep it straight.
◆ When you are both comfortable, ask your partner to gently extend your arms up and back. Hold and repeat exercise.

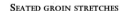

## HAMSTRING STRETCHES

MUSCLES WORKED:
HAMSTRINGS
HOLD: 8–30 SECONDS
GOOD FOR: RUNNING,
SWIMMING

## HAMSTRING STRETCHES

◆ Lie on your back on the floor with your partner kneeling beside you. Bend your right leg for support and raise your left leg, keeping it as straight as you can. Rest it against your partner's shoulder, so that his shoulder acts as a brace.

◆ When you are both comfortable, your partner should grip your left leg above the knee and ankle.

◆ When you are ready, ask your partner to push your left leg gently toward your chest.

◆ Stop when you feel mild tension. Release and repeat exercise using your other leg.

## LYING GROIN STRETCH

◆ Lie comfortably on the floor with your back straight, head in line with your spine and your abdominals pulled in. Bend your knees and rest your head on your arms.

◆ Your partner should now kneel astride your legs.

◆ Take a breath in, and as you breathe out, lift your head and shoulders up and twist your upper body to the left. As you do this, your partner should hold your calves to keep your feet flat on the floor. Hold. Repeat, twisting to the right.

## LYING GROIN STRETCH

MUSCLES WORKED:
ADDUCTORS, RECTUS
ABDOMINIS
HOLD: 10–30 SECONDS
GOOD FOR: CYCLING,
RUNNING, BASKETBALL

# JOINING A GYM OR HEALTH CLUB

*Before you join a gym or health club, consider whether it will suit your needs.*

## Ask yourself:

- [ ] Do I need special facilities and equipment?
- [ ] Is the gym in a convenient location?
- [ ] Do I need a gym all year round or for winter use only?
- [ ] Would I benefit from professional instruction from a trainer?
- [ ] Am I motivated enough to train by myself or do I need the atmosphere and stimulation of others to stay committed?
- [ ] Do I like team games?
- [ ] Will the guilt factor (paying and then not going) work in my favor?
- [ ] Can I afford the cost of a gym?

Many people who join a gym or health club somehow fail to keep up the momentum of going after the first few weeks or months. If this has happened to you in the past, be honest with yourself and draw up a list of what got in the way last time.

If you have already decided to opt for gym membership, do a bit of homework before committing yourself financially. Ask around among your friends and colleagues. They may be prepared to recommend their own club or gym, and they should be happy to tell you about any problems they may have encountered.

Visit the club on more than one occasion at the times you are likely to want to use the facilities. It would be good to see it during the week and at the busier times in the evenings and on the weekend, and to reassure yourself that you won't have to wait to use the equipment. Telephone to check the manner and knowledge of the reception staff, which is often a good indication of the general standards of a gym or club. There are various aspects you should consider when making your choice.

## STAFF

**Observation** Are there enough staff and are they easily identifiable; friendly; readily available; posers or there to help you; bored or active?

**Questions** Do the staff have recognized qualifications; regular training; personal experience; depth of knowledge through practice rather than theory (this may not be the case with new employees); do you feel intimidated by their looks/body shape; what is the average number of instructors; what is the staff turnover rate?

## EQUIPMENT

**Observation** Are there enough machines for the number of users; is there a variety of equipment; does it look of good quality and up to date; what are the floors made of (sprung wooden floors are better than concrete and carpet, for example)?

**Questions** How often is the equipment professionally cleaned and serviced; are materials (such as a cloth and spray) available for you to clean equipment before using it; is broken equipment repaired promptly?

## ENVIRONMENT

**Observation** Is the reception area welcoming; how busy is the club; is it well ventilated; is the lighting good; how much space has been set aside for a warm-up area; how high are the music levels; do you like the choice of music; are there obvious soda machines and water fountains; are there plenty of visible clocks with clear second hands so that you can time your activities; is there any evidence of smoking; can you tell that the shower areas are regularly cleaned; what are the changing facilities like; is the place generally clean and fresh?

**Questions** What are the security arrangements; what forms of insurance does the gym or club carry; is there a pleasant waiting/refreshment area for family and friends to use; can you play a personal stereo?

## SERVICES

**Observation** What general and safety information is on view; are free magazines displayed for use by members; can you look into the therapy rooms; is the safety equipment (such as oxygen cylinders, masks, and first aid kits) clearly visible; how big is the swimming pool, if any; is there a jacuzzi and/or sauna available; is there a nursery?

**Questions** What do you get for your basic membership fee (for example, fitness testing); what extras do you have to pay for; is medical screening offered; are you personally monitored while exercising; is there ongoing assessment of your progress; is therapy available on site; is there a member of staff always on duty who is fully trained in cardiopulmonary resuscitation; can you attend classes/workshops for members; what is the maximum number of people allowed in any one class?

**General questions** What are the costs; are there any discounts offered (such as family membership schemes); can you take temporary membership until you are completely satisfied with the facilities offered; can you pay by installments; do you have to join or can you pay at each visit; how convenient is the gym for home/work; who else do you know who uses it; is it privately run or part of a city complex; can you take a friend; what are the hours; what other facilities are offered (such as massage or physiotherapy)?

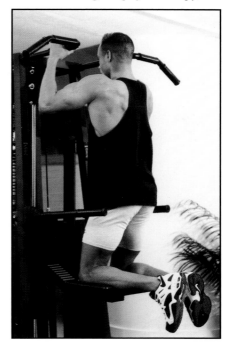

# WARM UP

*A warm-up routine is an integral part of any exercise program and should never be shortened or considered unnecessary.*

Between 10 and 15 minutes is the minimum time you should allow to prepare your body systems for action. A good warm-up routine will:
◆ improve the function of your cardiovascular system
◆ help your muscles to contract more efficiently
◆ increase your flexibility
◆ raise your pulse rate from resting to 40–60 percent of its maximum
◆ increase the flow of synovial fluid to make your joints pliable
◆ reduce the risk of injury.

Perform all warm-up exercises in a slow, smooth, and balanced way, using actions that are similar to your intended routine. Include rhythmic exercises, such as swinging and rotating movements, and static exercises, such as stretching and reaching movements. Count each movement so you don't overdo any particular one.

The temperature of the warm-up environment should be cool rather than cold. Start off wearing adequate layers of clothing, particularly if you are exercising outdoors. As you become warmer, remove a layer of clothing at a time. Try to start your main program immediately after you have finished your warm-up routine. If this is not possible for some reason, put any clothing you may have taken off while warming up back on and check how your body feels before starting your routine.

Choose a series of movements from the options below and right. Remember to check your pulse rate occasionally (*see pp. 10–11*) until you get to know the "feel" of your own body.

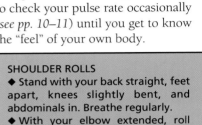

**SHOULDER ROLLS**
◆ Stand with your back straight, feet apart, knees slightly bent, and abdominals in. Breathe regularly.
◆ With your elbow extended, roll one shoulder in a clockwise and then a counterclockwise direction.
◆ Repeat this with your other shoulder and then with both together. Repeat all movements 5–10 times.

**SHOULDER ROLLS**
GOOD FOR: BACK, LEGS, ARMS, STOMACH

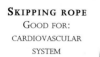

**SKIPPING ROPE**
GOOD FOR:
CARDIOVASCULAR
SYSTEM

## SKIPPING ROPE

◆ Use a jump rope with ball-bearing handles or a speed rope for a better action. Keep your movements light; try not to pound the ground too hard.

◆ Hold the rope in a comfortable grip with your arms extended to the sides and the rope behind you.

◆ Skip for 1 minute and then rest and repeat. Increase the skipping time to 5 minutes.

◆ Vary the routine with different leg movements. If you have never skipped before, it is natural to jump over the rope with both feet together. As your coordination improves, introduce rocking jumps – stepping over the rope with the same leading foot. Change your leading foot halfway through.

**ARM SWINGS**
GOOD FOR: BACK,
LEGS, ARMS,
STOMACH

## ARM SWINGS

◆ Stand with your legs more than shoulder width apart, knees bent, arms relaxed, and hands crossed at the front of your body.

◆ Inhale deeply as you swing your arms above your head in a wide outward sweep and straighten your legs.

◆ As you exhale, return your arms to the start position and bend your knees.

◆ Repeat exercise 5–10 times.

# COOL DOWN

*It is all too easy to dismiss the benefits of cooling down, especially if you are feeling tired and the shower is the place you most want to be.*

A good cooling-down routine is widely accepted as being one way of alleviating stiffness and helping to bring your body systems back to normal levels. The exercises used for cooling down are similar to those for warming up (*see pp. 26–27*), or you could try the two-stage routine described below. Stage one slows down your cardiovascular system, while Stage two assists in the removal of waste products from your body.

**Stage one**  Gently jog in place for about 4 minutes; then walk in place for another minute.

**Stage two**  Use a range of static stretching exercises, such as the two shown here, that most closely relate to the muscles used in your main training session. Do them for about 5 minutes.

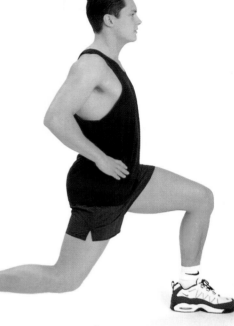

**LUNGES**
GOOD FOR: THIGHS, BUTTOCKS

**YOU WILL INCREASE YOUR RISK OF INJURY IF YOU:**

◆ allow too little time to warm up and cool down
◆ have poor technique (check with a trainer if you are unsure)
◆ use faulty equipment or shoes
◆ exercise too intensely
◆ do not rest for 24 hours between strenuous workouts
◆ attempt activities that do not suit your body type
◆ eat a poor diet
◆ ignore advice from trainers
◆ exercise after drinking alcohol.

**LUNGES**
◆ Stand with your feet comfortably apart, legs slightly bent, back straight, pelvis forward, and abdominals in. Place your hands on your hips, inhale, and step forward with your left foot.
◆ Keeping your body aligned centrally, bend your front knee and drop your back knee toward the ground. Stop as you feel tension. Hold for 8–10 seconds.
◆ Exhale as you lift back to a standing position, pushing with your heel.
◆ Repeat 5–10 times with each leg.

## CAT STRETCHES
◆ Kneel on the ground with your back straight, head and spine aligned, and hands stretched in front of you. Breathe regularly.
◆ Gently lower your body to the ground, pushing your arms forward until you feel tension in the shoulders. Hold for 8–10 seconds. Repeat 5–10 times.

**CAT STRETCHES**
GOOD FOR: SHOULDERS, SIDES

| COMMON INJURIES | REMEDY |
|---|---|
| **Acute injury** | In the short term, think RICE – Rest, Ice, Compression, and Elevation. Seek advice from a doctor or a sports injury clinic. |
| **Back pain** | Ease off on strenuous exercise. Start gentle exercises to strengthen and support back and abdominal muscles (swimming is good). |
| **Blisters** | Wash with soap and water and dry with a clean cotton pad; cover with a bandage. |
| **Heat exhaustion** | (This occurs in hot, humid weather and is the result of dehydration.) Lie down in the shade or a cool room. Elevate legs to increase the blood supply to the brain. Replace fluids using a solution of 1 tsp salt per quart of water. Drink as much as you comfortably can. |
| **Joint pain or swelling** | Ease off on exercising. You could also try using cushioned insoles in your shoes. |
| **Sore muscles** | Rest within the session or allow 24–48 hours between intense exercise. Cut back on strenuous exercise or concentrate on other areas. Continue with gentle exercise. Use adequate warm-up and cool-down routines. |
| **Strained muscles** | This is more acute than general soreness, but treated in the same way. If a particular area remains tender, check with your trainer. |
| **Sore tendons** | Treat as for sore/strained muscles. Always warm up properly and wear good-quality shoes that fit and support. Check the work surface – avoid concrete and unsprung floors. |

# THE ELEMENTS OF F

*Your body evolved to cope with a high level of activity, but the chances are that in modern times you have developed into a "couch potato." Inactivity encourages sluggish metabolism, weight gain, high blood pressure, high blood cholesterol levels, and poor digestion. With a little hard work, however, you can boost your metabolic rate, tone your muscles, and generally feel more energized.*

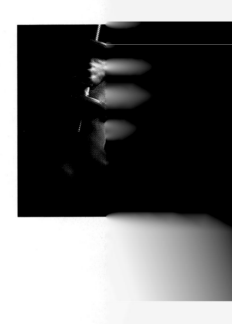

**Is exercise safe?** If you have not exercised recently, don't run to the squash court right off the bat. Plan your program sensibly and build up gradually. That way, you will feel good without taking unnecessary risks. If you have a medical problem, such as a heart condition, check with your doctor before starting.

◆ Avoid exercising for at least two hours after a heavy meal.
◆ Don't drink any alcohol for at least six hours before your workout.
◆ Warm up and cool down properly.
◆ Take plenty of fluids.
◆ Wear the correct clothing (*see p. 21*).
◆ Stop if you get dizzy, nauseous, or very short of breath, or if you break out into a cold sweat or feel any pain.

**Indoors or out?** Exercising indoors may be easier to arrange, but studies have shown that exercising outdoors gets you fitter more quickly. So even if you prefer to work out indoors, try to be outdoors occasionally.

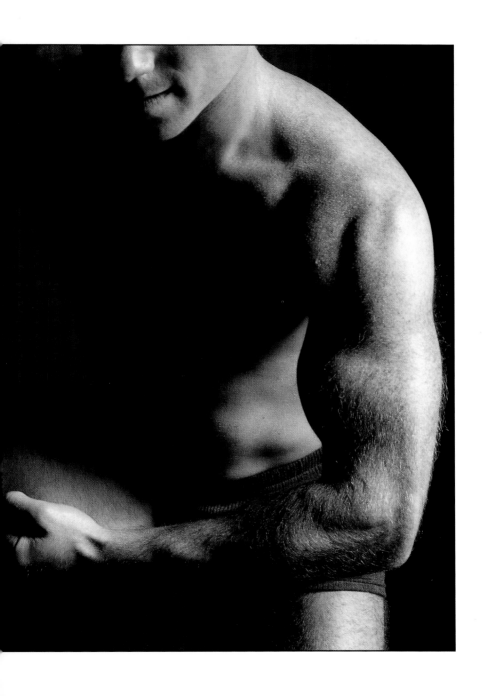

# ENERGY FOR MOVEMENT

*The "fuel" your body uses for movement is chemical energy, stored in the muscles or dissolved in the blood, and has to be converted into mechanical energy for use.*

The bodily processes that are involved in converting chemical energy into mechanical energy are fairly inefficient, since most of it (about 80 percent) is released as heat. This is why you feel hot when exercising.

Carbohydrates (contained in sugars and starches) and fats are the fuels that power this energy-conversion cycle. Another vital component is oxygen; indeed, oxygen is necessary for any activity that continues for longer than about three minutes. If oxygen is not available in a muscle because, say, you have used it in a quick burst of aerobic activity such as sprinting, extra energy is taken from your ATP stores (*see p. 16*). Your ability to sustain such anaerobic work therefore depends on how great these stores are.

Anaerobic action also results in an oxygen "debt" which must be "repaid" later during a period of rest – your breathing rate remains raised until this has been done. Aerobic activity, by contrast, delivers oxygen immediately via the blood supply and uses body fat stores as part of its fuel supply. This is why aerobic activity (together with a controlled diet) is so important in a weight-loss program.

Your cardiovascular system responds to this activity in three ways to increase the flow of blood: your blood vessels dilate, your heart rate increases, and blood is diverted from your internal body organs to supply the muscles and to the skin to cool your body down.

## EXERCISE AND STAMINA, SUPPLENESS AND STRENGTH

Studies have found that if you are active you are less likely to become ill or obese in later life, since participating in even moderately vigorous sports can significantly reduce the risk of death from heart disease. Exercises that increase stamina benefit your heart in particular, but this is only one element of fitness. Strong muscles and supple joints are also vital. The table opposite shows the way different sports affect the three S's, but remember that the amount of effort you put into an activity makes a big difference to what you get out of it. Your efforts will help you to:

◆ Burn calories to reduce weight. Brisk walking for about 30 minutes each day uses up 200 calories – enough to lose one pound every two weeks.

◆ Remove cholesterol from your arteries and reduce the clogging process.

◆ Reduce your blood pressure (it rises during exercise to take extra blood to the muscles, but your resting rate will be lower as a result).

◆ Reduce your stress levels (non-competitive sports, such as swimming and walking, lower epiniphrine and other stress hormones and stimulate production of endorphin, sometimes called the pleasure hormone).

◆ Reduce your dependence on smoking and alcohol.

◆ Improve your sexual performance.

◆ Add to the quality of your life.

# HEALTH BENEFITS OF DIFFERENT SPORTS

| Activity | Stamina | Suppleness | Strength |
|---|---|---|---|
| Aerobics | ▲▲▲ | ▲▲▲ | ▲▲ |
| American football | ▲▲▲ | ▲▲▲ | ▲▲▲ |
| Badminton | ▲▲ | ▲▲▲ | ▲▲ |
| Baseball | ▲▲ | ▲ | ▲▲ |
| Basketball | ▲▲▲ | ▲▲▲ | ▲▲▲ |
| Bicycling | ▲▲▲▲ | ▲▲ | ▲▲▲ |
| Circuit training | ▲▲▲ | ▲▲▲ | ▲▲▲ |
| Golf | ▲ | ▲▲▲ | ▲ |
| Jogging | ▲▲▲▲ | ▲▲ | ▲▲ |
| Karate/judo | ▲ | ▲▲ | ▲ |
| Skiing (downhill) | ▲▲ | ▲▲ | ▲▲ |
| Skipping rope | ▲▲▲ | ▲▲ | ▲▲ |
| Soccer | ▲▲▲ | ▲▲▲ | ▲▲▲ |
| Squash | ▲▲▲ | ▲▲▲ | ▲▲ |
| Swimming (hard) | ▲▲▲▲ | ▲▲▲▲ | ▲▲▲▲ |
| Tennis | ▲▲ | ▲▲▲ | ▲▲ |
| Track and field | ▲▲▲ | ▲▲ | ▲▲▲ |
| Walking (gentle) | ▲▲ | ▲ | ▲ |
| Walking (brisk) | ▲▲▲ | ▲ | ▲▲ |
| Weight training | ▲ | ▲▲▲ | ▲ |
| Yoga | ▲ | ▲▲▲ | ▲ |

KEY ▲ Slight effect    ▲▲▲ Beneficial effect
▲▲ Moderate effect    ▲▲▲▲ Excellent effect

# STAMINA

*Stamina helps you to keep going without becoming too short of breath or feeling pain in your muscles.*

You should be able to climb a flight of stairs or run for a bus without feeling physically distressed. Improving your stamina, and hence, the efficiency of your cardiovascular system, will enable you to cope more easily with prolonged exertion. In the short term, exercising for stamina will allow you to be active for longer periods and put in greater effort without exhausting yourself. In the long term, it helps to protect you against heart disease. In particular, the exercises designed for stamina are intended to increase heart volume and contractile force (which means that more blood is pumped per beat). This in turn improves the blood supply to the heart muscle, sending extra oxygen to all your muscles. Increasing your stamina also boosts your muscle energy stores, or ATP levels (*see p. 16*), and improves both your aerobic and anaerobic capacities. For maximum benefit from these exercises, repeat them between 12 and 40 times, depending on your fitness level.

## STAMINA ◆ *Running and jogging*

*Affordable and satisfying, running and jogging can be a part of any daily routine.*

These two activities are closely related, and the demands they make on the body are much the same. They require similar exercises, training, and techniques. Both start with a heel-first motion, and the body becomes slightly airborne as you push off with the ball of the foot and the stride lengthens. Good posture is important for both. Keep upright and allow your chest to expand. Develop a rhythmic action which uses a high knee movement and relaxed swinging arms. Use gentle jogging – either outside or on the spot indoors – as part of warm-up and cool-down routines for other sports (*see pp. 26-29*).

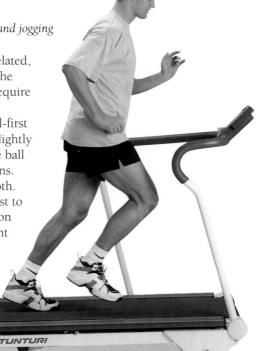

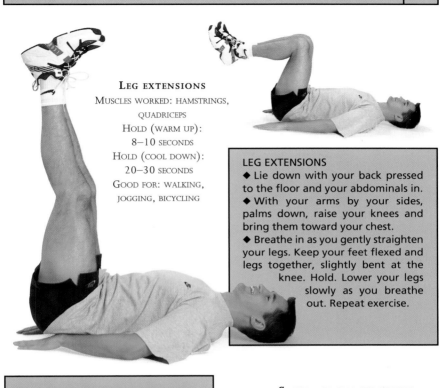

## Leg extensions

Muscles worked: hamstrings, quadriceps
Hold (warm up): 8–10 seconds
Hold (cool down): 20–30 seconds
Good for: walking, jogging, bicycling

### LEG EXTENSIONS
◆ Lie down with your back pressed to the floor and your abdominals in.
◆ With your arms by your sides, palms down, raise your knees and bring them toward your chest.
◆ Breathe in as you gently straighten your legs. Keep your feet flexed and legs together, slightly bent at the knee. Hold. Lower your legs slowly as you breathe out. Repeat exercise.

### SEATED GROIN STRETCHES
◆ Sit with your back straight, head in line with your spine, legs apart, and abdominals in.
◆ Rest your hands on your upper thighs. Keep your body upright and lift and move forward from the hips, putting your hands flat on the floor in front of you.
◆ Reach forward from the lower back area until you feel slight tension in the groin, lower back, and the backs of your legs. Hold. Repeat exercise.

### Seated groin stretches
Muscles worked: hamstrings, adductors, erector spinae
Hold (warm up): 8–10 seconds
Hold (cool down): 20–30 seconds
Good for: walking, running, rowing

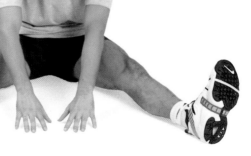

## STAMINA ◆ *Brisk walking*

*An entirely natural form of exercise, walking is great for*
*relieving stress and tension.*

Walking is enjoyable as a solitary activity, with a companion, or even at a club, and requires no expensive equipment unless you intend to take it up competitively. If you have problems with high-impact sports, such as jogging or running, then walking is particularly valuable.

Brisk walking, which must be distinguished from simply ambling, is excellent in terms of stamina, but it does not score so highly for suppleness or strength. So, to achieve all-round fitness, you need to combine brisk walking with other exercises. It is a particularly good starter activity for everybody or for older men who wish to remain fit and active.

Beginners should strive to walk 1 mile (1.5 km) in about 20 minutes, increasing to 3 miles (5 km) in about 50 minutes after 10 weeks. Try to walk at least 3 times a week, but short, brisk walks of at least 10 minutes each day are just as good. You should still be able to maintain a normal conversation while walking at a brisk pace.

If you intend to walk (or jog) as a form of exercise, the correct technique is important. You will naturally have your own personal style, but four general rules apply to everybody:

**Stride length** This must suit your height and leg length. Don't try to match the stride of someone who is much taller than you.

**Pace** The faster you move, the more weight you should transfer to your toes; the slower you move, the more you will use the flat of your feet. Try to use the ground as a springboard to ease you into the next stride and to develop an easy, rhythmic movement.

**Posture** The correct posture makes you more mechanically efficient. Try to walk or jog upright with a comfortably straight back.

**Relaxation** The more tense you are, the harder your body has to work. A good warm-up routine (*see pp. 26-27*) will help to relax your muscles.

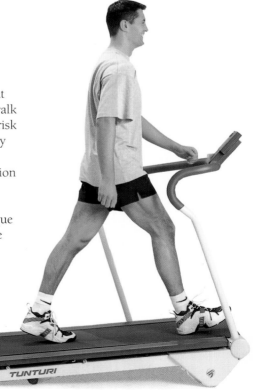

## STANDING CALF STRETCHES
◆ Stand with your back straight, your head in line with your spine, pelvis tilted forward, and your abdominals in.
◆ With your hands on your left thigh, move your left foot slightly in front of your right. Keep the foot in line with your hip.
◆ Bend your knees to transfer weight toward your toes, keeping your pelvis forward. When you feel tension in the lower calf, hold. Repeat with your other leg.

### STANDING CALF STRETCHES
MUSCLES WORKED: SOLEUS, GASTROCNEMIUS
HOLD (WARM UP): 8–10 SECONDS
HOLD (COOL DOWN): 20–30 SECONDS
GOOD FOR: WALKING, BICYCLING, JOGGING

### STANDING GROIN STRETCHES
MUSCLES WORKED: QUADRICEPS, SARTORIUS
HOLD (WARM UP): 8–10 SECONDS
HOLD (COOL DOWN): 20–30 SECONDS
GOOD FOR: RUNNING, SWIMMING, BICYCLING

## STANDING GROIN STRETCHES
◆ Standing with a straight back and your feet hip width apart, take a large stride to the side with your left leg. Keep your other leg straight.
◆ Bend your left knee, turning your toes out 45 degrees.
◆ Keep your hips square and slowly press your weight down into your heels. Hold when you feel tension in the groin.
◆ Repeat exercise with your other leg.

# STAMINA ◆ *Bicycling*

*Using an exercise bicycle is an excellent all-weather activity for improving your overall fitness.*

In addition to being a good anaerobic exercise, bicycling also improves the efficiency of the cardiovascular system. In terms of suppleness and maintaining mobility, it is a particularly beneficial activity for older men. Bicycling concentrates on the lower torso and is not seen as a weight-bearing activity. However, it is good to include it in a cross-training program (*see pp. 74–76*). Using an exercise bicycle, it is possible to work out at home, in the gym, or at the office. A good-quality machine will be adjustable, allowing you to gradually build up your speed and air resistance.

At the start of your program, stay in low gear so that resistance is not too high and you can concentrate on pedaling technique and speed. As your stamina develops, begin to introduce short, intense bursts (30–60 seconds) in the middle and at the end of your session, increasing them as you become fitter.

### HAMSTRING CURLS
MUSCLES WORKED:
HAMSTRINGS, GLUTEUS
MAXIMUS
HOLD: 8–10 SECONDS
GOOD FOR: BICYCLING,
RUNNING, SWIMMING

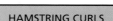

HAMSTRING CURLS
◆ Lie face down on the floor with your head resting on your right forearm and your left arm straight out. Keep your abdominals in.
◆ With your hips on the floor and knees together, raise your right knee 2 in (5 cm) off the ground with the foot flexed. Inhale.
◆ Gently curl your right foot toward your buttock, breathing out. Keep your hips on the floor. Hold. Breathe in as you slowly lower your leg back to within 2 in (5 cm) of the floor.
◆ Repeat exercise without putting your knee down. Repeat the sequence with your other leg.

# STAMINA ◆ *Rowing*

*For an exercise that uses all the major muscle groups, rowing is ideal.*

If you want to improve your aerobic fitness, rowing is a good exercise to choose. It is also an anaerobic exercise, since the short, intense bursts of activity increase your tolerance to lactic acid build-up in the muscles. Because all of the major muscle groups are involved, rowing is an ideal exercise to include in a cross-training program (*see pp 74-76*). And if you use a rowing machine, you can exercise year round – at the gym or at home, or even in the office.

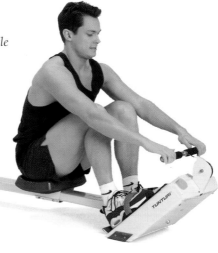

The correct posture and technique are important if you are to avoid lower back strain. If you are a beginner, seek professional advice from a trainer before you start. Always sit with your back straight and abdominals pulled in and maintain a smooth, continuous action. Start with about 10 strokes a minute and build up by adjusting the resistance of the machine as your aerobic efficiency improves.

### ABDOMINAL CRUNCHES
◆ Lie on your back with your knees bent, legs apart, and feet flat on the floor. Keep your lower back pressed to the floor and abdominals in.
◆ Put your hands on your thighs, head and spine aligned, and inhale.
◆ As you exhale, gently raise your head and shoulders, moving your hands toward your knees. Keep your lower back on the floor and make sure that your head and spine are still aligned. Hold the position.
◆ Breathe in again as you lower yourself gently to the floor.
◆ Repeat exercise as soon as your shoulders touch the floor, without relaxing your abdominals.

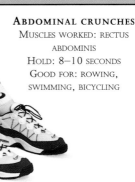

**ABDOMINAL CRUNCHES**
MUSCLES WORKED: RECTUS
ABDOMINIS
HOLD: 8–10 SECONDS
GOOD FOR: ROWING,
SWIMMING, BICYCLING

## STAMINA ◆ *Swimming*

*Often described as the perfect fitness activity, swimming combines stamina, suppleness, and strength.*

This exercise is ideal as part of a year-round fitness program, and if you swim with a partner, you could always introduce a competitive element. To increase your level of fitness even more, include some poolside exercises.

If you have a back problem but you don't want it to get in the way of your exercise routine, then swimming may be the answer, since the water helps to support your body weight.

There are four main strokes to practice for all-round benefit.

**Front crawl** The water should be at the mid-forehead level. With your legs slightly bent at the knee, kick constantly. Turn your head to alternate sides to breathe on every third arm stroke.

**Breast stroke** Your arms and your legs should look symmetrical and work simultaneously. Most of the power of this stroke comes from the kicking movement. Hold the extended arm and leg movement in order to improve the glide action. Keep the water at the mid-forehead level. Lift your head to breathe as you draw your arms back.

**Backstroke** Rest your back and head on the water and tuck your chin in. Exhale as one arm enters the water and inhale as the other does. Kick from your hips and try not to break the surface of the water with your knees or feet.

**Butterfly** Keep your feet together and kick once as your hands enter the water and once again as they leave it. Keep your shoulders level with the water's surface. Every second stroke, raise your head as your arms enter the water, breathe at the same time.

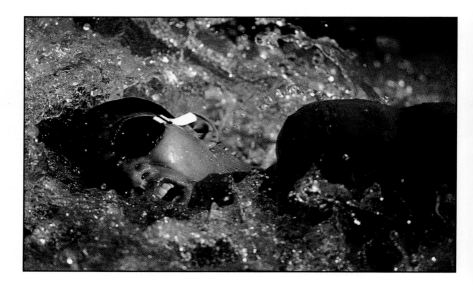

## TECHNIQUE

Concentrate on the following points
to improve your style for all strokes:

**Body position** This affects the whole
stroke, so (with the exception of the
breast stroke) your body should be
streamlined – as if swimming through
a tunnel. Keep your arms and legs
straight to help you move through
the water with minimal resistance.

**Leg action** Leg kicks help to maintain
a good body position. Kick as strongly
as possible to stay horizontal, but try
to minimize splashing.

**Arm action** Most of the power in a
stroke (except breast stroke) comes from
your arms. For maximum efficiency,
arm stroke should be disciplined.

**Breathing** Poor breathing technique
affects your swimming style. Try to
breathe regularly without interrupting
your arm and leg action.

**Timing** Aim to increase your distance
rather than your speed, since this allows
you to improve your technique and
build up stamina. Don't slow down as
you become fitter – you need to keep
your heart rate up for 20–30 minutes.

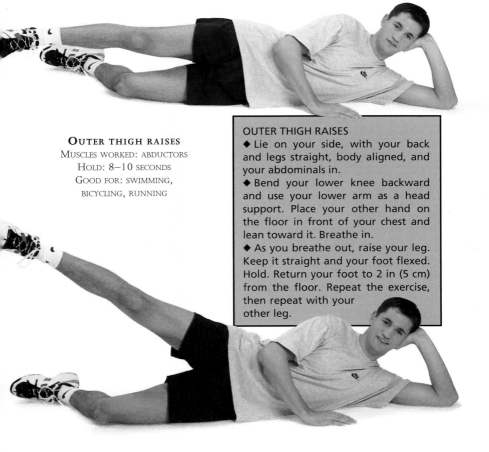

**OUTER THIGH RAISES**
MUSCLES WORKED: ABDUCTORS
HOLD: 8–10 SECONDS
GOOD FOR: SWIMMING,
BICYCLING, RUNNING

OUTER THIGH RAISES
◆ Lie on your side, with your back
and legs straight, body aligned, and
your abdominals in.
◆ Bend your lower knee backward
and use your lower arm as a head
support. Place your other hand on
the floor in front of your chest and
lean toward it. Breathe in.
◆ As you breathe out, raise your leg.
Keep it straight and your foot flexed.
Hold. Return your foot to 2 in (5 cm)
from the floor. Repeat the exercise,
then repeat with your
other leg.

# STRENGTH

*The ability to push, pull, and lift objects without effort requires strength.*

This element of a fitness program involves building up the muscle power and endurance needed for most sporting activities. To increase strength, you must exert force against a resistance, such as dumbbells or an exercise machine (at home, a can of beans makes an ideal improvised weight). You develop muscle tone (endurance) by reducing the weight factor and increasing the speed of the lift.

Do not launch into a weight-training program without some planning. An instructor will assist you in a gym; at home, start with light weights and build up resistance until you feel challenged. Injuries are often caused by using heavy weights before you are ready. To achieve maximum strength in each group of muscles, repeat an exercise between 6 and 12 times. As you improve, introduce sets of repetitions until you are repeating each set up to 6 times, with a short break between each.

Never train alone using heavy weights. Work with a partner who can take the weights from you if necessary. Belts should not be needed if you are using light weights as part of an all-round fitness program.

## STRENGTH ◆ *Legs*

MUSCLE GROUPS: *adductors, abductors, hamstrings, quadriceps, gastrocnemius, soleus, tibialis anterior*

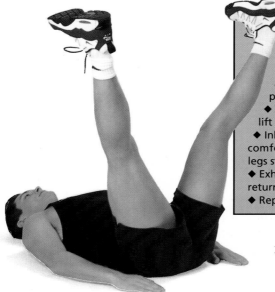

INNER THIGH RAISES
◆ Lie on your back with your lower back pressed to the floor, your head and shoulders relaxed, and your arms comfortably at your sides, palms down.
◆ Tighten your abdominals and lift your legs with the toes flexed.
◆ Inhale and open your legs to a comfortable position. Keep your legs straight. Hold the position.
◆ Exhale, slowly close your legs, and return to the starting position.
◆ Repeat exercise.

INNER THIGH RAISES
MUSCLES WORKED: ADDUCTORS
HOLD: 8–10 SECONDS
GOOD FOR: SWIMMING,
WEIGHT LIFTING

## PLIE SQUATS

◆ Dead-lift a dumbbell (*see p. 44*), holding it at the front of your body. Keep your back straight, pelvis forward, and abdominals in.

◆ Place your feet a little more than shoulder width apart, facing the front. Relax your shoulders.

◆ Inhale and slowly squat, bending at the knee and hip. Keep the dumbbell close to your body and do not drop below seat height.

◆ While exhaling, slowly rise to a standing position. Keep your heels on the floor. Pause and repeat the exercise.

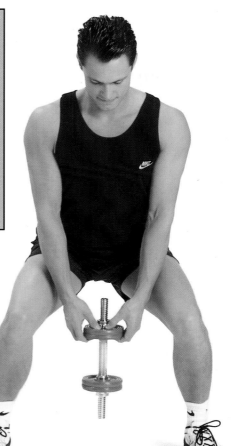

**PLIE SQUATS**
MUSCLES WORKED: QUADRICEPS,
HAMSTRINGS, GLUTEALS
HOLD: CONTINUOUS MOVEMENT
GOOD FOR: CIRCUIT
TRAINING, BICYCLING

## HAMSTRING CURLS

◆ Lie face down with your head in the crook of your right arm, left arm extended, hips pressed down, and abdominals in.

◆ Heel first, lift your right leg until the knee is 2 in (5 cm) off the ground. Hold and inhale.

◆ As you exhale, curl your foot toward your buttocks, keeping your hips on the floor.

◆ Hold, inhale, and lower your leg until it is 2 in (5 cm) off the floor.

◆ Repeat the exercise with your left leg.

**HAMSTRING CURLS**
MUSCLES WORKED: HAMSTRINGS,
GLUTEUS MAXIMUS
HOLD: 8–10 SECONDS
GOOD FOR: BICYCLING,
RUNNING, SWIMMING

## HOW TO DEAD-LIFT
◆ Stand with your feet hip width apart and a pair of dumbbells on the floor on the outside of and at right angles to them. With a straight back, abdominals in, and pelvis forward, bend at the hips and knees and place your forearms on your knees.
◆ Lean forward, keeping your head and spine aligned. Take an overhand grip on the dumbbells and inhale.
◆ As you exhale, straighten your legs and stand, using your legs to lift the dumbbells to thigh height.
◆ To dead-lift a barbell, stand centered on the weight and continue as above.

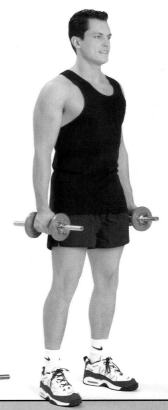

### BARBELL LUNGES
MUSCLES WORKED:
QUADRICEPS, HAMSTRINGS, GLUTEALS
HOLD: CONTINUOUS MOVEMENT
GOOD FOR: CIRCUIT TRAINING, ROWING

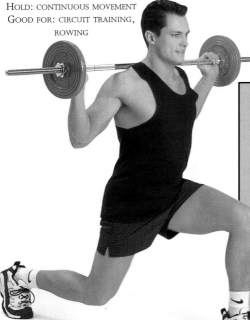

## BARBELL LUNGES
◆ Dead-lift a barbell to the height of your thighs.
◆ Flex your knees, press the bar over your head and lower it gently to your shoulders. Widen your grip on the bar for more control.
◆ Keeping your feet hip width apart, inhale and take a large step forward so that your back knee just brushes the ground.
◆ As you exhale, bring your front leg back and stand upright.
◆ Repeat with your other leg.
◆ To finish, narrow your grip on the bar, raise it above your head, and lower it gently to the floor. Do not use too heavy a weight or your technique will suffer.

## LEG EXTENSIONS

◆ Use an ankle weight suitable for your ability. Fasten it securely.
◆ Sit on a bench facing forward with the backs of your knees touching the bench. Keep your back straight and your abdominals in.
◆ Grip the bench behind, close to your buttocks. Inhale.
◆ As you exhale, raise your right leg with your toes pointing up and your knees together. Hold.
◆ Breathe in and then exhale as you lower your leg, holding about 2 in (5 cm) from the floor before touching down. Repeat exercise with the left leg.

**LEG EXTENSIONS**
MUSCLES WORKED:
QUADRICEPS
HOLD: 8–10 SECONDS
GOOD FOR: BICYCLING,
CIRCUIT TRAINING

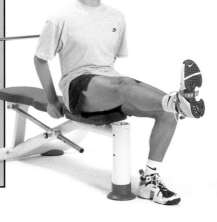

**SQUATS**
MUSCLES WORKED:
QUADRICEPS, HAMSTRINGS,
GLUTEALS
HOLD: CONTINUOUS
MOVEMENT
GOOD FOR: BICYCLING, ROWING

## SQUATS

◆ Dead-lift a barbell to the height of your thighs. Keep a straight back, abdominals in, pelvis forward, and chest raised.
◆ With your feet facing forward more than hip width apart, bend your knees, lift the bar above your head, and lower it behind your head to your shoulders.
◆ Inhale, bend at the knees and hips, and squat down no lower than seat height.
◆ Keep the weight over your ankles, and your back straight.
◆ Exhale and slowly stand up.
◆ To finish, narrow your grip on the bar and lower it gently to the floor.

# STRENGTH ◆ *Arms*

MUSCLE GROUPS: *biceps brachii, triceps, brachialis, brachioradials*

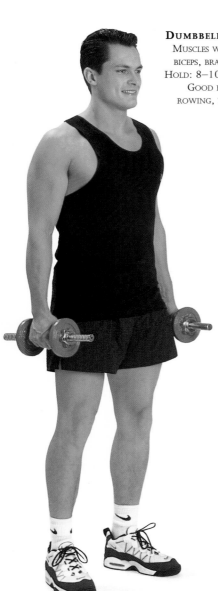

**DUMBBELL CURLS**
MUSCLES WORKED:
BICEPS, BRACHIALIS
HOLD: 8–10 SECONDS
GOOD FOR:
ROWING, TENNIS

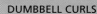

**DUMBBELL CURLS**
◆ Dead-lift a dumbbell in each hand (*see p. 44*).
◆ Stand with your feet comfortably apart and knees slightly bent.
◆ Keep your back straight, arms close to your body, and wrists straight. Inhale.
◆ As you exhale, raise each dumbbell in turn to shoulder level, twisting the dumbbell through 90 degrees. Hold.
◆ Lower the dumbbells while breathing in. Repeat exercise.

## LYING ELBOW EXTENSIONS

◆ Dead-lift a barbell (*see p. 44*) and hold it at thigh level. Sit on a bench with the weight in your lap.

◆ Lie back comfortably and place both feet on the floor or on the end of the bench. Keep your back flat and your abdominals in.

◆ Grip the barbell and extend your arms upward.

◆ As you inhale, lower the bar behind your head. Hold.

◆ As you exhale, return to the arm-extended position, keeping your elbows straight. Repeat exercise.

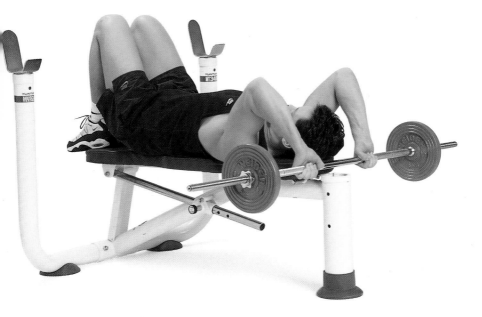

**LYING ELBOW EXTENSIONS**
MUSCLES WORKED:
TRICEPS
HOLD: 8–10 SECONDS
GOOD FOR: ROWING, WEIGHT
TRAINING, SWIMMING

## SEATED TRICEPS EXTENSIONS
MUSCLES WORKED: TRICEPS
HOLD: 8–10 SECONDS
GOOD FOR: ROWING, TENNIS

### SEATED TRICEPS EXTENSIONS
◆ Sit astride a bench with your feet flat, back straight, and your abdominals in. Dead-lift a dumbbell (see p. 44) in your right hand.
◆ Place your left hand on your knee and slowly lift the dumbbell to shoulder height. Pause and then straighten your arm above your head.
◆ As you inhale, take the dumbbell behind your shoulder blades, close to your body.
◆ Exhale as you reverse the weight through the same sequence. Repeat exercise.

## TRICEPS DIPS
MUSCLES WORKED: TRICEPS
HOLD: 8–10 SECONDS
GOOD FOR: SWIMMING, SQUASH, WEIGHT TRAINING

### TRICEPS DIPS
◆ Sit on the side of a bench with one hand at each side of your body. Keeping your back straight, abdominals in, and body aligned, ease yourself forward.
◆ Extend your legs forward. Keep your feet hip width apart.
◆ Inhale as you lower yourself as far as you can. Keep your back straight and close to the bench. Hold.
◆ Exhale as you return to the start position. Repeat exercise.

## STANDING TRICEPS EXTENSIONS
MUSCLES USED: TRICEPS
HOLD: CONTINUOUS EXERCISE
GOOD FOR: ROWING, TENNIS

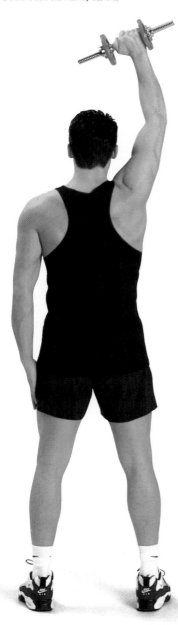

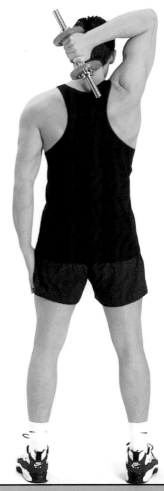

STANDING TRICEPS EXTENSIONS
◆ This is the same exercise in principle as the seated triceps extensions (opposite), except that it has more effect on the back.
◆ Stand with your feet facing forward and comfortably apart, back straight, body aligned, and abdominals in.
◆ Leave your free hand by your side throughout.
◆ Follow the instructions opposite. Repeat the exercise with both arms.

# STRENGTH ◆ *Chest*

MUSCLE GROUPS: *pectorals, serratus anterior*

### PUSH-UPS – BEGINNER
MUSCLES WORKED: ANTERIOR
DELTOIDS, PECTORALS, TRICEPS
HOLD: 8–10 SECONDS
GOOD FOR: SWIMMING, TENNIS,
WEIGHT TRAINING

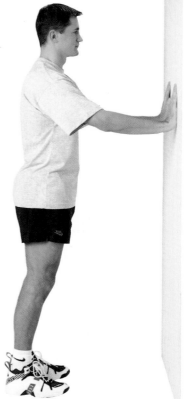

## PUSH-UPS – BEGINNER
◆ Stand facing a wall with your feet comfortably apart, pelvis forward, back straight, and abdominals in.
◆ Put your palms flat on the wall and level with your shoulders. Keep your body straight.
◆ Inhale and, keeping your back straight, lean toward your hands until your nose just touches the wall. Hold.
◆ Exhale and return to the upright position. Repeat exercise.

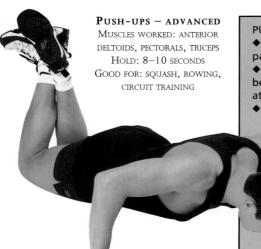

### PUSH-UPS – ADVANCED
MUSCLES WORKED: ANTERIOR
DELTOIDS, PECTORALS, TRICEPS
HOLD: 8–10 SECONDS
GOOD FOR: SQUASH, ROWING,
CIRCUIT TRAINING

## PUSH-UPS – ADVANCED
◆ Lie face down, elbows bent, and palms flat on the floor.
◆ With your knees hip width apart, bend your knees and cross your feet at the ankles.
◆ Lift your feet and lean forward so that your weight is over your hands.
◆ Inhale and, as you exhale, push up with your arms without locking your elbows. Keep your back straight throughout. Hold.
◆ Inhale and lower your chest to the floor. Repeat without a break.

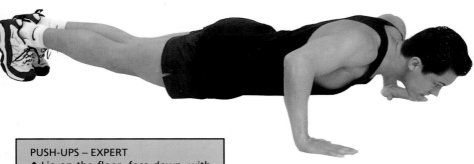

## PUSH-UPS – EXPERT
◆ Lie on the floor, face down, with your body in a straight line.
◆ Place your palms on the floor, 12 in (30 cm) to each side of your shoulders. Keep your back flat and abdominals in.
◆ Push up with your toes and hands to raise your chest off the ground.
◆ Inhale and lower your body until your chest touches the ground. Hold.
◆ Exhale and push back up.
◆ Keep your back straight and do not lock your elbow joints. Repeat exercise without a break.

**PUSH-UPS – EXPERT**
MUSCLES WORKED: PECTORALS, ANTERIOR DELTOIDS, TRICEPS
HOLD: 8–10 SECONDS
GOOD FOR: SWIMMING, ROWING, WEIGHT TRAINING

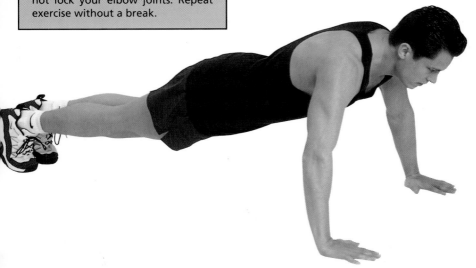

## STRENGTH ◆ *Neck, back, and shoulders*

Muscle groups: *sternocleidomastoid, trapezius, rhomboids, deltoids, teres major and minor, latissimus dorsi, erector spinae*

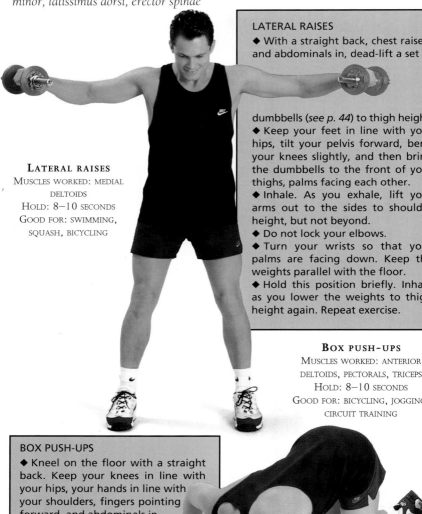

### LATERAL RAISES
◆ With a straight back, chest raised, and abdominals in, dead-lift a set of

**LATERAL RAISES**
Muscles worked: medial
deltoids
Hold: 8–10 seconds
Good for: swimming,
squash, bicycling

dumbbells (*see p. 44*) to thigh height.
◆ Keep your feet in line with your hips, tilt your pelvis forward, bend your knees slightly, and then bring the dumbbells to the front of your thighs, palms facing each other.
◆ Inhale. As you exhale, lift your arms out to the sides to shoulder height, but not beyond.
◆ Do not lock your elbows.
◆ Turn your wrists so that your palms are facing down. Keep the weights parallel with the floor.
◆ Hold this position briefly. Inhale as you lower the weights to thigh height again. Repeat exercise.

**Box push-ups**
Muscles worked: anterior
deltoids, pectorals, triceps
Hold: 8–10 seconds
Good for: bicycling, jogging,
circuit training

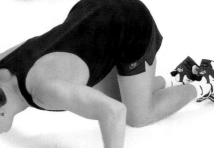

### BOX PUSH-UPS
◆ Kneel on the floor with a straight back. Keep your knees in line with your hips, your hands in line with your shoulders, fingers pointing forward, and abdominals in.
◆ As you inhale, bend your elbows and move your upper body forward until your nose touches the ground. Hold.
◆ Exhale as you return to a kneeling position. Repeat exercise.

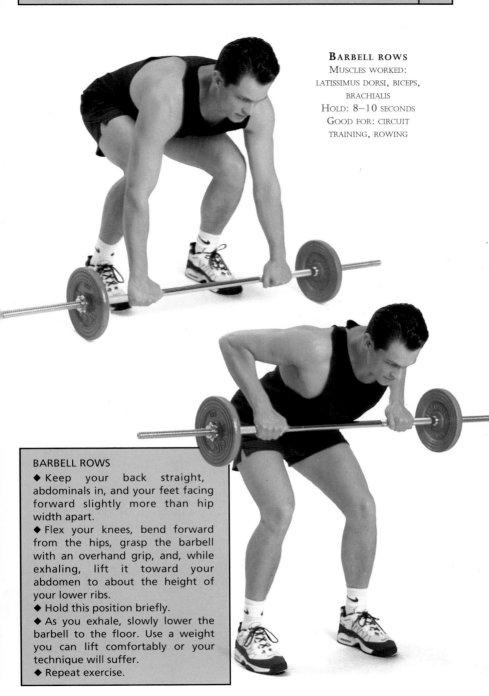

**BARBELL ROWS**
MUSCLES WORKED:
LATISSIMUS DORSI, BICEPS,
BRACHIALIS
HOLD: 8–10 SECONDS
GOOD FOR: CIRCUIT
TRAINING, ROWING

BARBELL ROWS
◆ Keep your back straight, abdominals in, and your feet facing forward slightly more than hip width apart.
◆ Flex your knees, bend forward from the hips, grasp the barbell with an overhand grip, and, while exhaling, lift it toward your abdomen to about the height of your lower ribs.
◆ Hold this position briefly.
◆ As you exhale, slowly lower the barbell to the floor. Use a weight you can lift comfortably or your technique will suffer.
◆ Repeat exercise.

## STRENGTH ◆ *Abdomen*
MUSCLE GROUPS: *rectus abdominis, external and internal obliques, lower pelvic muscles*

LOWER ABDOMINAL RAISES
◆ Lie on the floor on your back with your legs together, knees slightly bent, lower back pressed down flat to the floor, and your abdominals in.
◆ Cross your feet at the ankles.
◆ Place your arms comfortably at your sides, palms facing the floor, and inhale.
◆ As you exhale, gently raise your knees toward your chest, making sure you don't rock your body. Keep your abdominal muscles tight. Hold this position.
◆ Breathe in as you return to the floor position. Repeat exercise.

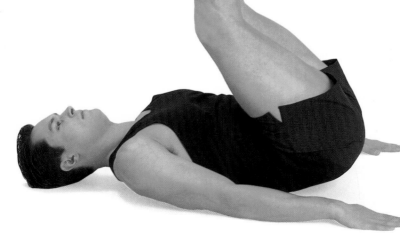

LOWER ABDOMINAL RAISES
MUSCLES WORKED:
LOWER PELVIC
HOLD: 8–10 SECONDS
GOOD FOR: ROWING, BICYCLING,
SWIMMING

## SINGLE ARM CRUNCHES
MUSCLES WORKED:
RECTUS ABDOMINIS
HOLD: 8–10 SECONDS
GOOD FOR: ROWING,
BICYCLING, SWIMMING

## SINGLE ARM CRUNCHES
◆ Lie on your back with your lower back pressed to the floor, feet flat, knees apart, and abdominals in.
◆ Put your left hand on your left thigh. Place your right hand under your head. Inhale.
◆ As you exhale, raise your shoulders and slide your left hand toward your knee. Do not move your right elbow forward. Hold.
◆ Breathe in as you lower your shoulders. Do not relax your abdominals.
◆ Repeat before your shoulders reach the floor. Repeat on your other side.

## TWISTS
◆ Lie on your back, knees bent, feet flat on the floor, lower back pressed down, and abdominals in.
◆ Place your hands behind your head. Rest your head in your hands with your elbows pulled back.
◆ Bring your left ankle up to rest on your right knee and inhale.
◆ As you exhale, raise your right shoulder up toward your left knee, twisting from the waist.
◆ Keep your lower back touching the floor. Hold.
◆ Inhale as you gently return to the flat position, keeping your abdominals tight. Repeat exercise.

## TWISTS
MUSCLES WORKED: EXTERNAL
OBLIQUES
HOLD: 8–10 SECONDS
GOOD FOR: BICYCLING, WEIGHT
TRAINING, ROWING

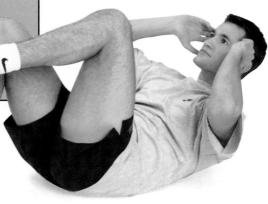

# SUPPLENESS

*Being supple means you can bend, stretch, and twist without discomfort or difficulty.*

Frequency, not intensity, is the key to success here. Perform a variety of muscle-stretching exercises regularly, and you will improve your range of joint movements and make the ligaments and tendons more flexible.

When planning your program, concentrate on the shoulders, lower back, hips, and legs. Stretching forms a vital part of any warm-up and cool-down routine (*see pp. 26–29*) and must complement any strengthening program, which shortens and tightens muscles. Stretching is also an energizer in the home, office, or when traveling.

It may take several weeks to feel any improvement. A flexible body is less prone to aches, and regular stretching improves posture and reduces the risk of injury and back problems.

**STRETCH SAFELY**
◆ Wear loose-fitting clothing.
◆ Warm up with rhythmic exercise before beginning your stretch routine (*see pp. 26–27*).
◆ Stretch until you feel tension and hold; 8–10 seconds maintains muscle length, 20–30 seconds increases muscle length.
◆ Never force a stretch until it hurts.
◆ Stretch smoothly. Don't jerk to try to increase the length of a stretch.
◆ Music with a strong beat encourages jerky, damaging movements, so it should be avoided.
◆ Always stretch muscles equally on both sides.
◆ Start your routine gently and repeat each exercise 8 to 12 times.
◆ If you experience any problems, slow down or stop.

## SUPPLENESS ◆ *Legs*

MUSCLE GROUPS: *quadriceps, hamstrings, gastrocnemius, soleus, adductors, abductors, tibialis anterior*

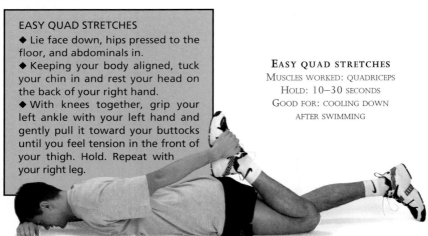

**EASY QUAD STRETCHES**
◆ Lie face down, hips pressed to the floor, and abdominals in.
◆ Keeping your body aligned, tuck your chin in and rest your head on the back of your right hand.
◆ With knees together, grip your left ankle with your left hand and gently pull it toward your buttocks until you feel tension in the front of your thigh. Hold. Repeat with your right leg.

EASY QUAD STRETCHES
MUSCLES WORKED: QUADRICEPS
HOLD: 10–30 SECONDS
GOOD FOR: COOLING DOWN
AFTER SWIMMING

## UPPER CALF STRETCHES

◆ Stand with a straight back, pelvis forward, feet comfortably apart, toes forward, and abdominals in.
◆ Use a chair back to help you balance if necessary. Step back with your right leg.
◆ Keeping your body aligned, bend your left knee and move your body weight over your left ankle.
◆ Press your right heel into the ground and feel the tension in your calf. Hold. Repeat exercise.

**UPPER CALF STRETCHES**
MUSCLES WORKED:
GASTROCNEMIUS
HOLD: 8–30 SECONDS
GOOD FOR: COOLING DOWN
AFTER BICYCLING

**SIDEWAYS QUAD STRETCHES**
MUSCLES WORKED: QUADRICEPS
HOLD: 8–30 SECONDS
GOOD FOR: WARMING UP
BEFORE SWIMMING, BICYCLING

## SIDEWAYS QUAD STRETCHES

◆ Lie on your right side with a straight back and abdominals in.
◆ Support your head in the palm of your right hand.
◆ If your body starts to rock, steady yourself by slightly bending your right knee.
◆ Bend your left leg toward your buttocks, using your left hand to increase the stretch.
◆ Hold when you feel tension in your left thigh. Repeat the exercise using your right leg.

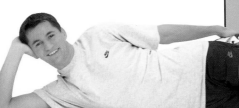

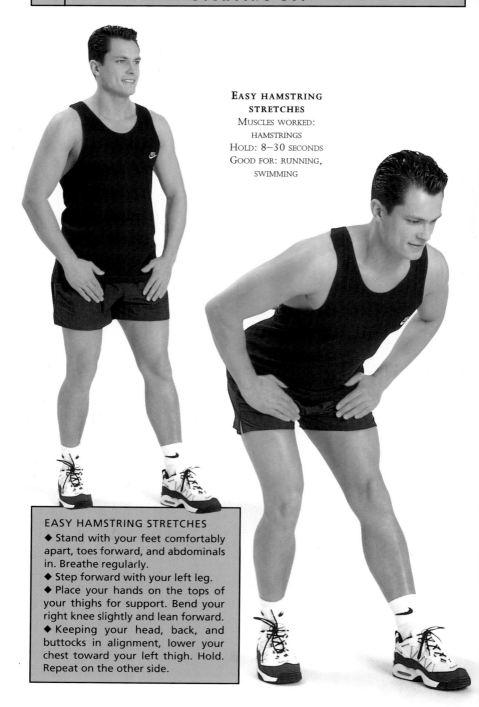

### EASY HAMSTRING STRETCHES

MUSCLES WORKED:
HAMSTRINGS
HOLD: 8–30 SECONDS
GOOD FOR: RUNNING,
SWIMMING

### EASY HAMSTRING STRETCHES

◆ Stand with your feet comfortably apart, toes forward, and abdominals in. Breathe regularly.
◆ Step forward with your left leg.
◆ Place your hands on the tops of your thighs for support. Bend your right knee slightly and lean forward.
◆ Keeping your head, back, and buttocks in alignment, lower your chest toward your left thigh. Hold. Repeat on the other side.

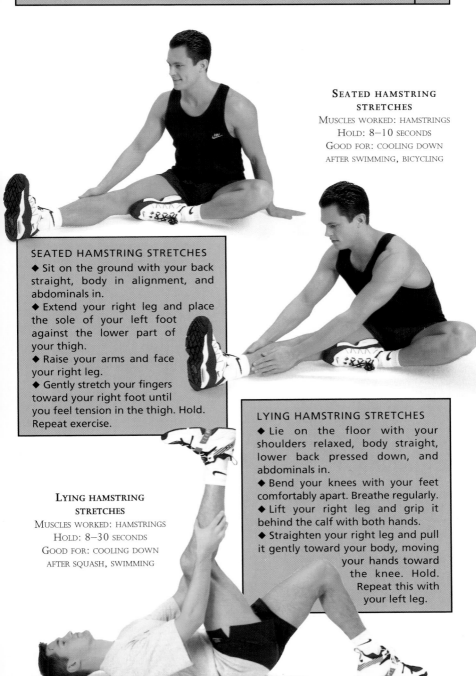

### SEATED HAMSTRING STRETCHES
MUSCLES WORKED: HAMSTRINGS
HOLD: 8–10 SECONDS
GOOD FOR: COOLING DOWN
AFTER SWIMMING, BICYCLING

### SEATED HAMSTRING STRETCHES
◆ Sit on the ground with your back straight, body in alignment, and abdominals in.
◆ Extend your right leg and place the sole of your left foot against the lower part of your thigh.
◆ Raise your arms and face your right leg.
◆ Gently stretch your fingers toward your right foot until you feel tension in the thigh. Hold. Repeat exercise.

### LYING HAMSTRING STRETCHES
◆ Lie on the floor with your shoulders relaxed, body straight, lower back pressed down, and abdominals in.
◆ Bend your knees with your feet comfortably apart. Breathe regularly.
◆ Lift your right leg and grip it behind the calf with both hands.
◆ Straighten your right leg and pull it gently toward your body, moving your hands toward the knee. Hold. Repeat this with your left leg.

### LYING HAMSTRING STRETCHES
MUSCLES WORKED: HAMSTRINGS
HOLD: 8–30 SECONDS
GOOD FOR: COOLING DOWN
AFTER SQUASH, SWIMMING

## SUPPLENESS ✦ *Arms, chest, and neck*

*Muscle groups: sternocleidomastoid, pectorals, serratus anterior, brachialis, triceps, biceps, brachio-radialis*

### TRICEPS STRETCHES
MUSCLES WORKED: TRICEPS, ANTERIOR DELTOIDS
HOLD: 8–30 SECONDS
GOOD FOR: COOLING DOWN AFTER
TENNIS

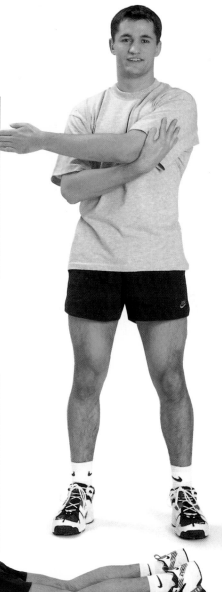

**TRICEPS STRETCHES**
◆ Stand with your feet comfortably apart. Keep your knees slightly bent, pelvis forward, back straight, and abdominals in.
◆ Breathe regularly throughout.
◆ Hold your left arm across your chest and put your right hand on your upper arm.
◆ Gently stretch your left arm across your chest.
◆ Hold. Repeat exercise with your other arm.

### CHEST RAISES
MUSCLES WORKED: PECTORALS
HOLD: 8–30 SECONDS
GOOD FOR: WARMING UP BEFORE
TENNIS, WEIGHT TRAINING
(AFTER RHYTHMIC EXERCISES)

**CHEST RAISES**
◆ Lie on the floor with your pelvis flat, legs together, feet extended, and your abdominals in. Breathe regularly throughout.
◆ Lock your fingers together behind your back with elbows slightly bent.
◆ Raise your arms, pulling your shoulder blades together until you feel tension in the chest. Hold at that point. Repeat exercise.

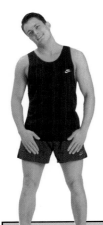

### NECK STRETCHES
MUSCLES WORKED:
STERNOCLEIDOMASTOIDS
HOLD: 8–10 SECONDS
GOOD FOR: WARMING
UP BEFORE SWIMMING
(AFTER RHYTHMIC
EXERCISES)

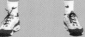

## NECK STRETCHES
◆ Stand with your feet comfortably apart. Keep your knees slightly bent, pelvis forward, back straight and abdominals in. Keep your body aligned centrally. Breathe regularly throughout.
◆ Keeping your shoulders level, gently move the right side of your head toward your right shoulder. Hold. Repeat on the other side.

## STANDING CHEST STRETCHES
◆ Stand with your feet comfortably apart, knees slightly bent, pelvis forward, back straight, hands on hips, and abdominals in. Breathe regularly throughout.
◆ Keeping your body in alignment, move your hands back to rest on your buttocks and draw your shoulder blades together until you feel tension in your chest. Hold at that point. Repeat exercise.

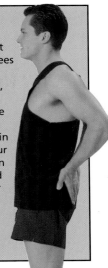

### STANDING CHEST STRETCHES
MUSCLES WORKED: PECTORALS
HOLD: 8–30 SECONDS
GOOD FOR: COOLING
DOWN AFTER
SWIMMING, ROWING

### FOREARM STRETCHES
MUSCLES WORKED: BRACHIALIS
HOLD: 8–10 SECONDS
GOOD FOR: WARMING UP BEFORE TENNIS, WEIGHT
TRAINING (AFTER RHYTHMIC EXERCISES)

## FOREARM STRETCHES
◆ Kneel with your body in alignment and your abdominals in. Breathe regularly throughout.
◆ Place your hands flat on the floor, aligned with your shoulders, with your fingers facing your knees.
◆ Lean backward with your body, hands flat, until you feel tension in your lower arms. Hold. Repeat exercise.

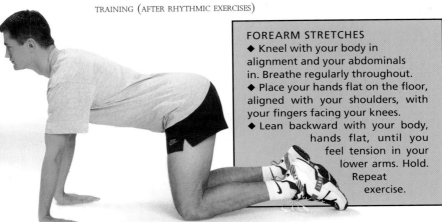

## SUPPLENESS ✦ *Back and shoulders*

MUSCLE GROUPS: *deltoids, teres major and minor, latissimus dorsi, trapezius*

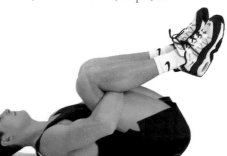

**BACK CURLS**
◆ Lie on your back with your knees drawn up to your chest in a tight curl.
◆ Keeping your head and spine in line, relax your neck, shoulders, and spine.
◆ Pull in your abdominals and aim for a good spine curve. Hold.
Repeat exercise.

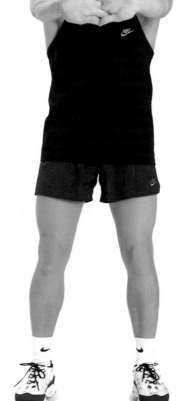

**BACK CURLS**
MUSCLES WORKED: ERECTOR SPINAE
HOLD: 8–30 SECONDS
GOOD FOR: COOLING DOWN AFTER
SWIMMING, ROWING

**OPEN BACK STRETCHES**
◆ Stand with your back straight, feet comfortably apart, pelvis forward, knees slightly bent, and your abdominals in. Breathe regularly throughout.
◆ Stretch out both of your arms in front of you at shoulder height and bend your elbows slightly.
◆ With your fingers locked securely together and with the backs of your hands facing your body, gently stretch your arms forward to open out your upper back. Hold. Repeat exercise.

**OPEN BACK STRETCHES**
MUSCLES WORKED: TRAPEZIUS, TRICEPS, RHOMBOIDS
HOLD: 8–30 SECONDS
GOOD FOR: COOLING DOWN AFTER
SWIMMING, TENNIS

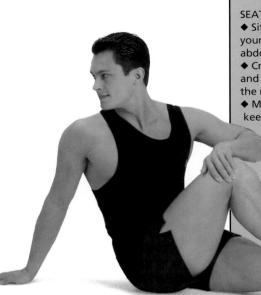

## SEATED BACK STRETCHES
◆ Sit on the floor with your hands at your sides, back straight, and your abdominals in.
◆ Cross your right leg over your left and place your foot flat on floor at the mid-calf level. Breathe regularly.
◆ Move your right hand backward, keeping it close to your body, and put your left hand on the outside of your right knee.
◆ Pull your right knee toward the mid-body and twist your upper body toward your right arm, looking back over your right shoulder. Keep your back straight. Hold when you feel tension. Repeat on the other side.

**SEATED BACK STRETCHES**
MUSCLES WORKED: ERECTOR SPINAE,
GLUTEALS, STERNOCLEIDOMASTOIDS,
ABDUCTORS
HOLD: 8–30 SECONDS
GOOD FOR: COOLING DOWN AFTER
ROWING, WEIGHT TRAINING

## LOWER BACK RAISES
◆ Lie face down with your pelvis forward, legs together, toes touching the ground, and abdominals in.
◆ Place your palms on your buttocks and inhale.
◆ As you exhale, lift your shoulders and head, keeping a smooth line. Hold when you feel tension.
◆ Lower your body while inhaling. Repeat exercise.

**LOWER BACK RAISES**
MUSCLES WORKED: ERECTOR SPINAE
HOLD: 8–10 SECONDS
GOOD FOR: ROWING, WEIGHT
TRAINING, BICYCLING

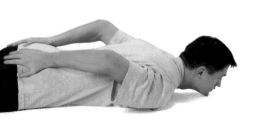

# SUPPLENESS ◆ *Hips and Buttocks*

MUSCLE GROUPS: *gluteus medius, gluteus maximus, sartorius*

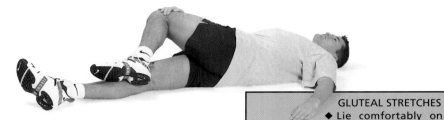

### GLUTEAL STRETCHES

MUSCLES WORKED: GLUTEUS
MAXIMUS

HOLD: 8–30 SECONDS

GOOD FOR: WARMING UP BEFORE
SWIMMING (AFTER RHYTHMIC
EXERCISES)

GLUTEAL STRETCHES
◆ Lie comfortably on the floor with your back pressed against the ground, body straight, and abdominals in.
◆ Breathe regularly throughout.
◆ Extend your left arm to the side, lift your left knee, and hold it with your right hand.
◆ Gently stretch your left knee across your right leg until you feel tension in the buttocks and hips.
◆ Hold. Repeat on both sides.

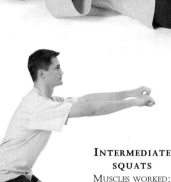

### INTERMEDIATE SQUATS

MUSCLES WORKED:
HAMSTRINGS, GLUTEALS,
QUADRICEPS

HOLD: CONTINUOUS
EXERCISE

GOOD FOR: SOCCER,
TENNIS, SQUASH
WEIGHT TRAINING

INTERMEDIATE SQUATS
◆ Stand with a straight back, pelvis tilted forward, and abdominals in.
◆ Inhale and bend from the knees and hips into a squatting position no lower than seat height.
◆ As you squat, extend your arms at shoulder height. Do not arch your back at any point. Keep your weight over your ankles. Hold.
◆ Exhale as you slowly stand up. Repeat exercise.

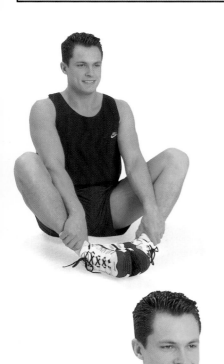

**SEATED INNER-THIGH STRETCHES**
MUSCLES WORKED: ADDUCTORS
HOLD: 8–30 SECONDS
GOOD FOR: WARMING UP BEFORE SWIMMING

### SEATED INNER-THIGH STRETCHES
◆ Sit comfortably on the floor with your knees drawn up. Keep your back straight, your head and body aligned, and your abdominals in.
◆ Align the soles of your feet and place them squarely together, and then allow your knees to fall naturally apart toward the floor.
◆ Place your hands on your lower calves just above the ankles and press your knees down gently with your elbows until you start to feel tension in your thighs.
◆ Hold. Repeat exercise.

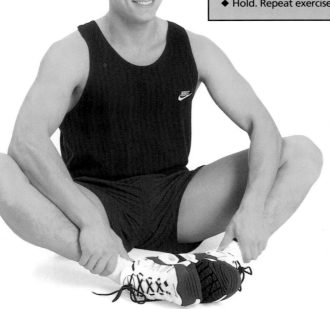

# SUPPLENESS ◆ *Abdomen*

MUSCLE GROUPS: *rectus abdominis, obliques*

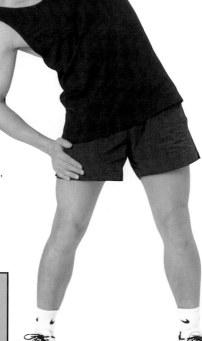

**STANDING SIDE STRETCHES**
MUSCLES WORKED: EXTERNAL OBLIQUES
HOLD: 8–30 SECONDS
GOOD FOR: WARMING UP OR COOLING DOWN

STANDING SIDE STRETCHES
◆ Stand in a wide squat position with your back straight, abdominals in, and your hips tilted forward.
◆ Place your right hand on your thigh.
◆ As you inhale, raise your left hand above your head. Do not lean forward or backward.
◆ Tilt your upper body to the right. Make sure you keep your head aligned with your spine.
◆ Hold as soon as you feel tension in your trunk and waist. Breathe regularly. Repeat exercise to the left.

**TOTAL BODY STRETCHES**
MUSCLES WORKED: RECTUS ABDOMINIS, OBLIQUES, TRAPEZIUS, QUADRICEPS, TRICEPS
HOLD: 8–30 SECONDS
GOOD FOR: WARMING UP OR COOLING DOWN

TOTAL BODY STRETCHES
◆ Lie on your back with your body straight, legs together, arms raised behind your head, lower back pushed down, and abdominals in.
◆ Inhale.
◆ As you exhale, stretch your arms and legs as far as you can. Breathe regularly and hold.
◆ Repeat exercise.

### THE SPHINX

◆ Lie face down with your nose touching the floor, body in alignment, and abdominals in.

◆ Place your hands and forearms in front of you, your hands level with your head. Inhale.

◆ As you exhale, gently lift your upper body and stretch forward from the abdominal area. Keep your head and back in alignment and your hips and arms on the ground. Breathe regularly and hold. Repeat exercise.

### THE SPHINX
MUSCLES WORKED: RECTUS ABDOMINIS
HOLD: 8–30 SECONDS
GOOD FOR: WARMING UP BEFORE WEIGHT TRAINING, ROWING

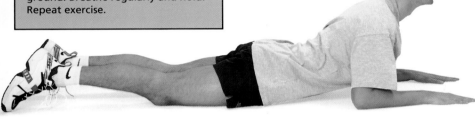

### SEATED SIDE STRETCHES
MUSCLES WORKED: EXTERNAL OBLIQUES
HOLD: 8–30 SECONDS
GOOD FOR: WARMING UP BEFORE ROWING, SWIMMING

### SEATED SIDE STRETCHES

◆ Sit comfortably on the floor with your legs crossed, knees bent, back straight, and abdominals in.

◆ Put your left hand on the floor to provide support and lift your right arm above your head.

◆ As you inhale, stretch your right hand and arm above and then over your head. Keep your buttocks firmly on the floor. Breathe regularly as you hold the stretch. Repeat exercise on the other side.

# CIRCUIT AND CROSS T

*Popular with modern athletes, both these forms of training maximize the three S's – stamina, suppleness, and strength – and allow you to plan your exercise routine from a wide choice of activities in order to gain maximum benefit with minimum risk.*

**Circuit training** You can follow a circuit-training program either at home or in the gym. Use it as a way of complementing other activities and to add variety to your exercise. The time factor is another great advantage of circuit training – you can complete a circuit in under an hour, including warming up and cooling down. Circuit training does not focus on suppleness, however, so if you intend to use it as your regular routine, you should include a variety of good stretching movements in your cool-down.

**Cross training** Originally, cross training was based on the theory that if you exercise one arm only, the other arm will also become stronger. It will not be as strong, but muscle growth will be stimulated in the unused limb. This is because of the proximity of nerve paths in the spinal region. Nowadays, the term cross training has a much wider meaning and is used to describe the way athletes exercise using a variety of sports to increase fitness. For example, a runner may cross train by using weights, and a swimmer can bicycle.

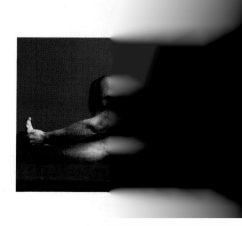

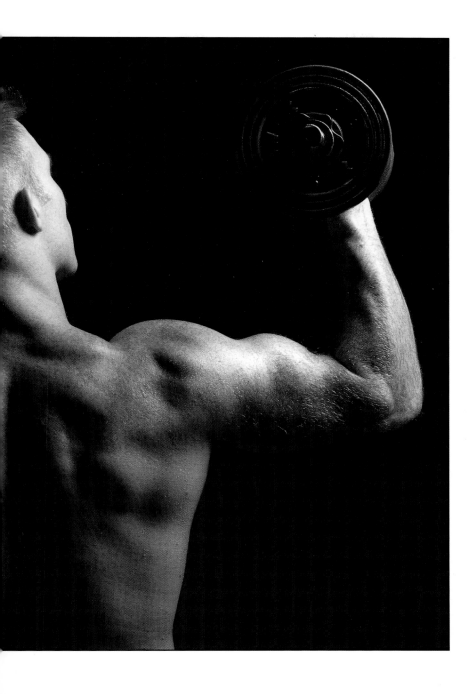

# CIRCUIT TRAINING

*At its simplest, circuit training is intense exercise interspersed with periods of rest.*

The theory behind circuit training is that benefits accrue more rapidly if several types of exercise are combined, because there is simultaneous improvement in four related physiological areas:
◆ Muscular strength
◆ Muscular endurance
◆ Aerobic power
◆ Energy combustion.
The types of exercises used in circuit training can vary (*see below and opposite*), as can the work-to-rest ratio. If you are a beginner, complete 1 circuit; if you are at intermediate level, complete between 2 and 3 circuits; if expert, between 3 and 5 circuits.

The body's voluntary muscles will gradually adapt to the increased activity and strengthen by being continually subjected to overload (repetition of an exercise). If you repeat an activity over and over, interspersed with short rests, "worked" areas become stronger and can repeat the action for longer, and with greater intensity, before tiring.

## DEVISING A CIRCUIT

Home and gym circuits are designed to work core muscle groups (*see pp. 72–73*). These, in turn, are helped by the muscle groups on the extremities. Work in a body, legs, body, legs sequence for strength exercises, to minimize the interaction of muscle groups, and to maximize the benefit of the rest period. Interspersing aerobic exercises helps to flush lactic acid from your system.

## RESISTANCE TRAINING

This type of training gives different results depending on how you exercise. Resistance work is built of repetitions, or "reps," and "sets" of exercises. A set is one group of exercises performed together and usually has between 12 and 40 reps, depending on your ability. For a balanced routine, aim toward working on each muscle group with two sets of exercise per workout.

## GYM CIRCUIT TRAINING

The principles of circuit training are the same wherever you work out. If you need some extra motivation to maintain your program, however, then a gym may be best for you.

A gym circuit has several other advantages over a home circuit: the attention of an expert; a choice of equipment; and an opportunity to increase your skills. As you progress, you can introduce weights into the program with less risk of injury under the guidance of an instructor.

## EXAMPLE OF A BASIC HOME CIRCUIT

| Strength | Aerobic | Strength | Aerobic | Strength | Aerobic |
|---|---|---|---|---|---|
| Body | Legs | Legs | Legs | Body | Legs |
| Push ups | Jump rope | Wall sits | Bicycling | Crunches | Burpees |
| 10–12 reps | 30–40 secs | 10–20 reps | 30–40 secs | 10–20 reps | 30–40 secs |

## BURPEES

◆ Crouch with your hands more than shoulder width apart in front of you. Keep your abdominals in and your head and spine aligned.
◆ Jump into the air, extending your arms above your head.
◆ Adopt the start position again and extend both legs behind you.
◆ Jump your legs forward toward the start position and leap back into the air. Repeat.

### BURPEES
MUSCLES WORKED:
HAMSTRINGS, QUADRICEPS, OBLIQUES
HOLD: CONTINUOUS MOVEMENT
GOOD FOR: AEROBIC TRAINING

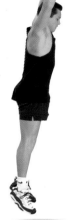
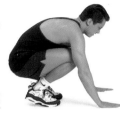

### WALL SITS
MUSCLES WORKED:
QUADRICEPS, HAMSTRINGS, GASTROCNEMIUS
HOLD: 20–60 SECONDS
GOOD FOR: WEIGHT TRAINING

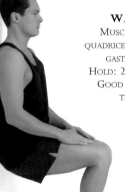

## WALL SITS

◆ Stand about 2 ft (60 cm) from a wall with your toes facing forward and your feet hip width apart.
◆ Bending at the knees and hips, press your lower back against the wall. Lower yourself this way until you reach a 90-degree angle at the hips – as if sitting on a chair.
◆ Hold the position for as long as it is comfortable, with your abdominals pulled in. Repeat.

### SQUAT THRUSTS
MUSCLES WORKED:
HAMSTRINGS, QUADRICEPS, BICEPS
HOLD: CONTINUOUS MOVEMENT
GOOD FOR: WEIGHT TRAINING

## SQUAT THRUSTS

◆ Crouch with your hands more than shoulder width apart. Keep your abdominals in and your head and spine aligned, and look down.
◆ Rise up on your toes and lift your buttocks. Keeping your left leg close to your chest, extend your right leg. Change legs rapidly.
◆ Repeat.

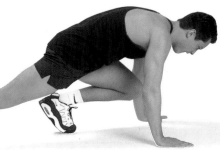

# GUIDELINES FOR TRAINING

◆ Include a variety of stations (activities), each specifically designed to increase strength or aerobic fitness.

◆ Create a balance of different activities to make sure that you achieve whole-body fitness.

◆ Alternate exercises so that you work your upper and lower body.

◆ Always work in a body, legs, body, legs order.

◆ Move quickly between stations in order to improve muscular strength, endurance, and aerobic fitness.

◆ If you are a beginner, rest for long enough to replace your ATP levels (see p. 16). It takes about 30 seconds to restore half of your ATP levels and about 2 minutes to restore them fully.

◆ Work complementary sets of muscles – for example, triceps/biceps, quadriceps/hamstrings.

◆ Introduce weights or machines to add variety to your circuit as you become more experienced.

◆ Good training means working to your personal limits, not to exhaustion.

◆ Concentrate on technique rather than on the speed of your circuit.

◆ If you are struggling to complete the circuits, lower the repetition load.

## EXAMPLES OF STRENGTH EXERCISES

| Home circuit | Muscles worked | Gym circuit |
| --- | --- | --- |
| wall push-ups | pectorals, latissimus dorsi | wall push-ups |
| crunches | abdominals | abdominal raises |
| leg extensions | quadriceps | leg extensions |
| lateral raises | deltoids, trapezius | lateral raises |
| hamstring curls | hamstrings | hamstring curls |
| floor push-ups | pectorals, triceps | bench presses |
| squats/lunges | quadriceps, hamstrings | leg squats |
| dumbbell curls | biceps | barbell rows |
| twists | external obliques | twists |
| wall sits | quadriceps · | squats |
| bicycling | rectus abdominis/ex obliques | bicycling |

## EXAMPLES OF AEROBIC EXERCISES

**All of these exercises are suitable for home or gym circuits**

◆ Jump rope ◆ Stepping ◆ Burpees ◆ Jogging in place ◆ Jumping jacks

◆ Static bicycling ◆ Static rowing ◆ Squat thrusts

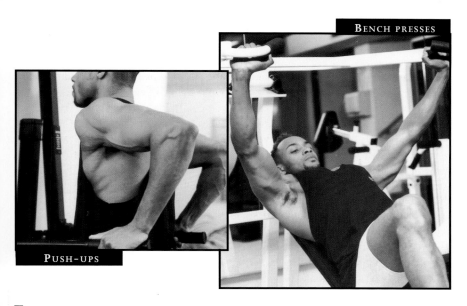

BENCH PRESSES

PUSH-UPS

## EXAMPLE OF A BASIC GYM CIRCUIT

| Strength | Aerobic | Strength | Aerobic | Strength | Aerobic |
|---|---|---|---|---|---|
| Body | Legs | Legs | Legs | Body | Legs |
| Bench press | Jump rope | Leg curl | Bicycling | Crunches | Stepping |
| 10–12 reps | 30–40 secs | 10–20 reps | 30–40 secs | 10–20 reps | 30–40 secs |

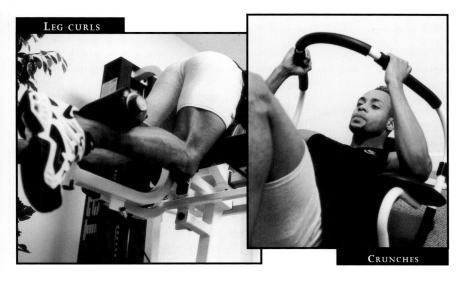

LEG CURLS

CRUNCHES

# CROSS TRAINING

*Combining a range of activities into a cross-training program creates a varied form of exercising that can be tailored to individual goals and objectives.*

If whole-body fitness is your objective, then a well-devised cross-training program could be perfect for you. This type of exercising is beneficial because each activity you include in your program works the major muscle groups (*see pp. 16–19*) in a slightly different way.

Cross training is also excellent if you want to lose weight and improve your body shape, since the more muscles you work, the more the complementary muscles play a part in burning calories. For example, as you work your biceps, your triceps are also brought into play,

so the overall benefit you derive is increased. A direct advantage of this is that as you exercise more of your muscle groups, you increase your body's capacity to process lactic acid, the waste product resulting from anaerobic activity that makes muscles feel heavy and sluggish.

By varying the time you spend on each activity, you can start to tailor your program to develop muscles in different ways. For example, if your fitness program is designed to help your skiing ability, then schedule more activities for lower body strength (such

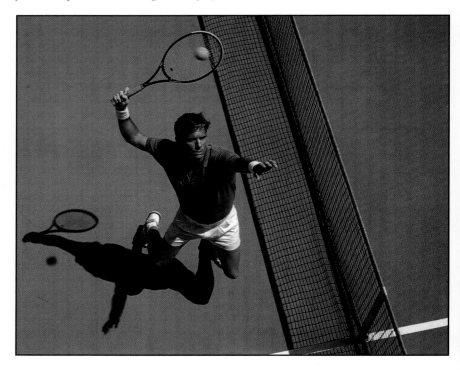

as push-ups, squats, and raises) and suppleness (whole body stretches and leg stretches).

Other advantages of cross training are that by planning a variety of activities, you can reduce the risk of overstraining any particular muscle group. Also, if you want some competition, you can combine your individual activities with team sports.

## DISADVANTAGES OF CROSS TRAINING

Most athletes would agree that there are few real disadvantages associated with cross training as a method of exercising. The most troublesome aspect probably involves getting your program of activities organized in the first place.

For cross training to be effective, however, you have to plan carefully to make sure that you include a balanced range of activities. Another potential drawback is that you must have access to a variety of sports. There may also be some additional expense if you need to buy equipment and accessories, such as rackets, shoes, or special clothing.

## DEVISING YOUR PROGRAM

The first step in planning a cross-training program is to explore the sports facilities in your local area that you could use on a regular basis. Less accessible sports, such as skiing or mountain climbing, could be included in a vacation plan. (Bear in mind that a cross-training program is not set in any way; you can alter it at will to suit new circumstances as they arise.) Then decide which of these activities are your favorites; which ones are

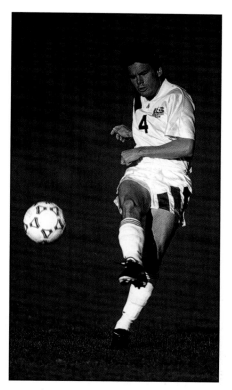

complementary to give a balanced range; which can be done at home; which need a club or gym facilities; and what you can afford.

To help you draw up this list, use the 10-week example plan and menu of activities on page 76 in conjunction with the stamina, suppleness, and strength rating table on page 33. The rules are few and simple:

◆ Include a combination of aerobic, general fitness, muscular strength, and muscular endurance exercises.
◆ Do not schedule sports that primarily use the same muscle group too close to each other.
◆ Leave a day for rest between very energetic sports.

# CROSS-TRAINING MENU AND ACTIVITY CHART

*From the first chart of menu options, choose activities from each of the four categories and adapt the 10-week activity plan from the second chart accordingly.*

| ACTIVITY BENEFIT | SPORT |
|---|---|
| Aerobic | stepping, jump rope, bicycling, brisk walking, running |
| Strength | circuit and weight training, hard swimming, martial arts |
| Endurance | rowing, jogging, running, swimming |
| General fitness | tennis, squash, basketball, volleyball, walking, swimming |

| 10-week plan | Monday | Wednesday | Friday | Sunday |
|---|---|---|---|---|
| Week 1 | bicycling | circuit | swimming | walking |
| Week 2 | step aerobics | rowing | walking | jump rope |
| Week 3 | running | basketball | circuit | swimming |
| Week 4 | bicycling | weights | tennis | rowing |
| Week 5 | jogging | martial arts | bicycling | squash |
| Week 6 | squash | swimming | walking | circuit |
| Week 7 | step aerobics | circuit | tennis | rowing |
| Week 8 | running | volleyball | rowing | bicycling |
| Week 9 | jump rope | rowing | circuit | walking |
| Week 10 | swimming | weights | bicycling | tennis |

# KEEP IT UP

*Make it fun, and keeping fit can become an enjoyable part of your daily routine.*

By this stage you should have achieved some of your goals – perhaps a leaner, healthier body, well-toned muscles, or a range of new interests. No doubt there will have been times when you have slipped back a little as your motivation flagged and other factors, both social and work-related, got in the way.

As you think about long-term exercise, remember the three S's – stamina, suppleness, and strength – and the important part they play in whole-body fitness. Review your reasons for starting to exercise in the first place, and if necessary, set yourself some new goals or try a different sports activity. Life is for enjoying right now, but the rest of your life is important, too, and it won't be half as much fun if you suffer from aches, pains, and stiffness every time you climb out of bed or run for a bus, let alone kick a ball around the park with your friends or children.

Whatever you have achieved up to this point will not remain a constant in the background, like a credit in the bank waiting to be drawn on at some later date when you need a bit of extra energy or strength. The slide from a peak of fitness to a breathless heap takes only a short time. Don't let it happen to you.

If you start to feel your motivation slipping, here are a few points that may inspire you to keep it up:

◆ Keep it simple – integrate your exercises into your daily routine, use a convenient gym or, if you exercise at home, don't do exercises that need complicated or expensive equipment.

◆ Exercise with a partner – you are far less likely to cancel.

◆ Change your exercise program on a regular basis – this will prevent boredom and keep your body from adapting to the same routine.

◆ Don't set unrealistic goals – small, weekly targets are easier to achieve.

◆ Don't become obsessive – exercise is supposed to be fun. It is not uncommon for people to become so single-minded about exercising that it gets in the way of the rest of their lives.

If you have followed the advice and practiced the exercises contained in this book, you will already feel different and know that physical activity is not a chore – it is fun and good for you!

# INDEX

Main mentions are in
**bold** type.

# ACKNOWLEDGMENTS

## PICTURE CREDITS

*All of the photographs in the book were taken by Laura Wickenden except for the following:*
p.40 Glyn Kirk/Tony Stone Images
p.74 Robert Harding Picture Library
p.75 The Image Bank
**Cover photography**: Paul Venning

*The publishers also wish to thank:*
**Models and fitness advisors:** Jason D. Boyce, Marcus K. White, Dave Green and Donovan H. Lewis
**Gym facilities:** Holmes Place, Barbican Health Club, 97 Aldergate Street, London, EC1A 4JR
**Clothes and shoes:** Worn throughout the exercises were all supplied by Nike
**Gym equipment:** B.M.I. UK/Distributor Bolton Stirland International: Rowing Machine p.39; Exercise Bike p.38; Weights Bench pp. 20, 45, 47, 48; Treadmill pp.34, 36.

**Author's acknowledgments:** Chris Leonard M.L.A.M, P.G. Dip., health and fitness manager at the Frank Lee Centre;
Addenbrooke's Hospital, Cambridge